Fasting Diet Book: A Complete Guide to Transform Your Health

Shawna Landry

Preface

Welcome to "Fasting Diet Book: A Complete Guide to Transform Your Health." This book is the culmination of my personal journey and deep passion for exploring the profound benefits of fasting.

Several years ago, I discovered fasting not just as a tool for weight management, but as a gateway to holistic health. As I delved deeper into the science behind fasting — its effects on metabolism, cellular rejuvenation, and mental clarity — I realized its potential to revolutionize how we approach wellness.

In this guide, I aim to demystify fasting, making it accessible to everyone regardless of their prior knowledge or experience. Whether you're curious about intermittent fasting, considering an extended fast, or seeking to integrate fasting with other health practices, this book offers a comprehensive roadmap.

Throughout these pages, you'll find evidence-based insights, practical tips for navigating challenges, and inspiring stories of individuals who have transformed their lives through fasting. From preparing for your first fast to maintaining long-term success, each chapter is designed to empower you on your journey to better health.

I invite you to explore, experiment, and discover the transformative power of fasting. Embrace this lifestyle with confidence, knowing that you have a wealth of knowledge and resources at your fingertips. Here's to embarking on a path towards vitality, clarity, and lasting well-being.

Warm regards,

Shawna Landry

Introduction: Embracing the Fasting Lifestyle

Welcome to "Fasting Diet Book: A Complete Guide to Transform Your Health." In the pages that follow, you will find a wealth of information, practical advice, and inspiration to help you embrace fasting as a powerful tool for enhancing your overall well-being.

My journey into the world of fasting began several years ago. Like many, I initially saw fasting as a means to shed a few pounds. However, as I delved deeper into the practice, I discovered that fasting offered far more than just weight loss. It became a gateway to improved mental clarity, increased energy, and a profound sense of balance in my life. This personal transformation inspired me to share the benefits of fasting with others.

Fasting is not a new concept. It has been practiced for centuries across various cultures and religions, often revered for its physical, mental, and spiritual benefits. Today, modern science is catching up, providing a wealth of evidence supporting the positive impacts of fasting on our health. From enhancing cellular repair processes to improving metabolic health and even potentially extending lifespan, fasting holds promise for anyone seeking to improve their health holistically.

This book is designed to guide you through the many facets of fasting. Whether you're a complete beginner or someone looking to refine and expand your fasting practice, you'll find comprehensive information tailored to your needs. We'll explore different types of fasting, delve into the science behind it, and discuss how to choose the right fasting method for your lifestyle and goals.

You'll also find practical advice on how to prepare for your first fast, navigate the challenges you might face, and safely break your fast. Additionally, we will look at how fasting can be customized for specific health goals, from weight loss and improved mental health to anti-aging and longevity.

In embracing the fasting lifestyle, it's essential to adopt a holistic approach. Fasting is not just about abstaining from food; it's about nourishing your body, mind, and spirit. This means making mindful choices about what you eat, how you think, and how you move your body. By integrating fasting with other healthy practices, you can maximize its benefits and create lasting positive changes in your life.

I invite you to join me on this transformative journey. Open yourself to the possibilities that fasting offers, and take the first step towards a healthier, more vibrant you. Whether your goal is to lose weight, gain mental clarity, or simply feel better in your own skin, this book will provide you with the tools and knowledge to achieve it.

Thank you for allowing me to be part of your journey. Let's embark on this path to health and vitality together.

Warm regards,

Shawna Landry

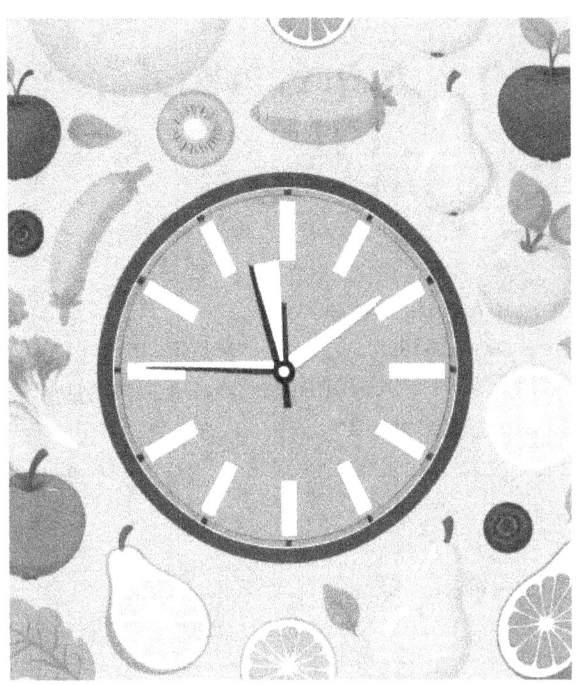

Chapter 1: Overview of the Benefits of Fasting

Fasting is more than just a dietary trend; it is a transformative practice with a myriad of health benefits that extend far beyond weight loss. In this chapter, we will explore the diverse and profound advantages of incorporating fasting into your lifestyle, backed by both ancient wisdom and modern scientific research.

1. Weight Loss and Fat Loss
One of the most popular reasons people turn to fasting is for weight management. By reducing the eating window, fasting can help lower overall calorie intake, leading to weight loss. Additionally, fasting promotes fat loss more effectively than conventional calorie restriction by enhancing the body's ability to burn fat for energy.

2. Improved Metabolic Health
Fasting has a significant impact on metabolic health. It can improve insulin sensitivity, lower blood sugar levels, and reduce insulin resistance, which are crucial factors in preventing and managing type 2 diabetes. Enhanced insulin sensitivity means your body can more effectively manage blood sugar levels, reducing the risk of metabolic syndrome and related conditions.

3. Enhanced Mental Clarity and Focus

Many people report improved mental clarity and focus during fasting periods. This is partly due to the reduction in blood sugar fluctuations and the increase in ketones, which serve as an efficient fuel source for the brain. Fasting can also promote the production of brain-derived neurotrophic factor (BDNF), a protein that supports brain health and cognitive function.

4. Longevity and Anti-Aging Effects
Fasting triggers a process called autophagy, where the body cleans out damaged cells and regenerates new ones. This cellular renewal process is linked to anti-aging benefits and longevity. By reducing oxidative stress and inflammation, fasting can slow down the aging process and extend lifespan.

5. Better Blood Sugar Control
Fasting helps stabilize blood sugar levels, preventing the spikes and crashes associated with frequent eating. This stability is particularly beneficial for individuals with or at risk of developing diabetes. Improved blood sugar control also translates to sustained energy levels and reduced cravings.

6. Reduced Inflammation and Improved Immune Function
Chronic inflammation is at the root of many diseases, including heart disease, cancer, and autoimmune conditions. Fasting can reduce inflammation markers in the body, thereby lowering the risk of chronic diseases. Moreover, fasting can enhance immune function by promoting the regeneration of immune cells, which boosts the body's ability to fight infections and illnesses.

7. Cardiovascular Health

Fasting has been shown to improve several key indicators of cardiovascular health, including blood pressure, cholesterol levels, and triglycerides. By reducing these risk factors, fasting can significantly lower the likelihood of developing heart disease.

8. Enhanced Hormone Regulation
Fasting influences the levels of several important hormones in the body. It increases the secretion of human growth hormone (HGH), which plays a role in muscle growth, metabolism, and overall health. Additionally, fasting helps regulate ghrelin (the hunger hormone) and leptin (the satiety hormone), which can help control appetite and promote a healthy weight.

9. Improved Gut Health
Intermittent fasting allows the digestive system to rest and repair. This can lead to improved gut health by enhancing the integrity of the gut lining and promoting a balanced microbiome. A healthy gut is essential for overall well-being, affecting everything from digestion to mental health.

10. Increased Energy and Physical Performance
Contrary to the belief that fasting leads to fatigue, many people experience increased energy levels and enhanced physical performance. Fasting can boost mitochondrial function and efficiency, which translates to better energy production and improved endurance during physical activities.

Conclusion
The benefits of fasting extend far beyond simple weight loss. From improved metabolic health and enhanced mental clarity to anti-aging effects and better immune function, fasting is a powerful tool for holistic health. By understanding and harnessing these benefits, you can transform your well-being and achieve a healthier, more vibrant life.

As we continue through this book, you'll gain deeper insights into the science behind these benefits, learn various fasting methods, and discover practical tips to integrate fasting into your daily routine. Embrace the fasting lifestyle and unlock your full potential for health and vitality.

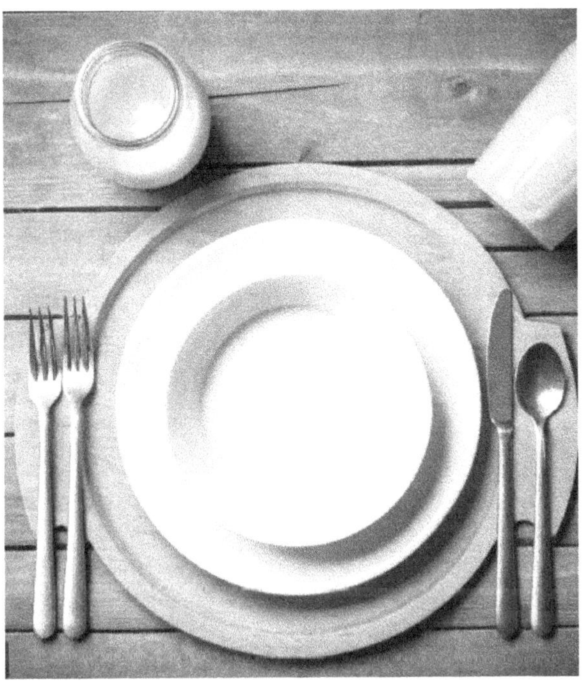

Chapter 2: The Importance of a Holistic Approach to Health

In today's fast-paced world, it's easy to become focused on quick fixes and single-solution strategies for health. However, achieving and maintaining optimal well-being requires a holistic approach—one that considers the interconnectedness of body, mind, and spirit. In this chapter, we will explore why a holistic perspective is crucial for effective health transformation and how fasting can be a central component of this approach.

Understanding Holistic Health
Holistic health emphasizes the whole person, not just specific symptoms or illnesses. It considers multiple facets of well-being, including physical health, mental clarity, emotional balance, and spiritual fulfillment. This integrative view recognizes that each aspect of health influences the others, creating a dynamic and interdependent system.

1. Physical Health
While fasting is often recognized for its physical benefits, such as weight loss and improved metabolic health, it should be combined with other healthy lifestyle practices for maximum impact. This includes:

Nutrition: Eating nutrient-dense, whole foods that provide essential vitamins and minerals.

Exercise: Engaging in regular physical activity to strengthen the body and improve cardiovascular health.

Sleep: Ensuring adequate rest and recovery through quality sleep, which is vital for overall health and healing.

2. Mental Health

Fasting can enhance mental clarity and focus, but its benefits are amplified when paired with practices that support mental health:

Mindfulness and Meditation: Techniques that promote relaxation and mental clarity, helping to reduce stress and improve cognitive function.

Stress Management: Strategies such as deep breathing, yoga, and time in nature to lower stress levels and support mental well-being.

Lifelong Learning: Engaging in activities that stimulate the mind and promote continuous learning and growth.

3. Emotional Health

Emotional well-being is critical for a balanced life and can be nurtured through:

Healthy Relationships: Building and maintaining supportive, positive relationships that provide emotional support.

Self-Reflection: Practices like journaling or therapy that help you understand and process your emotions.

Positive Mindset: Cultivating gratitude, resilience, and a positive outlook on life.

4. Spiritual Health

For many, spiritual health is a foundational aspect of overall well-being. It can be nurtured through:

Connection: Feeling connected to something larger than oneself, whether through religion, nature, or community.

Purpose: Identifying and pursuing one's purpose or passion in life.

Inner Peace: Practices like meditation, prayer, or contemplation that foster a sense of inner peace and balance.

The Synergy of a Holistic Approach

When fasting is integrated into a holistic health approach, the benefits of each practice are enhanced. For example:

Improved Nutrition: Fasting can help reset eating patterns and reduce cravings, making it easier to adopt a nutritious diet.

Enhanced Exercise: Combining fasting with physical activity can boost fat burning and improve physical performance.

Better Sleep: Fasting can regulate hormones that affect sleep, leading to more restful and restorative sleep.

Mental Resilience: The discipline and mindfulness developed through fasting can strengthen mental resilience and reduce stress.

Emotional Balance: By simplifying food choices and reducing emotional eating, fasting can help stabilize emotions.

Spiritual Growth: Many find that fasting enhances their spiritual practices, providing a deeper sense of connection and purpose.

Practical Tips for a Holistic Health Approach

Set Comprehensive Goals: Define health goals that encompass physical, mental, emotional, and spiritual well-being.

Create a Balanced Routine: Develop a daily routine that includes healthy eating, exercise, mindfulness, and time for self-care.

Listen to Your Body: Pay attention to how your body responds to fasting and other health practices, and adjust as needed.

Seek Support: Engage with communities, support groups, or professionals who can guide and encourage you on your holistic health journey.

Stay Flexible: Be open to modifying your approach as you learn more about what works best for your unique needs.
Conclusion
A holistic approach to health recognizes that true well-being is multifaceted, involving the integration of physical, mental, emotional, and spiritual health. Fasting, as a powerful tool within this framework, can enhance each of these areas when practiced thoughtfully and in combination with other healthy lifestyle choices. By embracing a holistic perspective, you can achieve deeper, more sustainable health transformation and a more vibrant, fulfilling life.

As we progress through this book, you'll learn more about how to effectively implement fasting within this broader context of holistic health, ensuring that you reap the maximum benefits for your body, mind, and spirit.

Chapter 3: Understanding Fasting

Fasting, an age-old practice, has gained renewed interest in recent years due to its profound health benefits. To fully appreciate its potential, it's essential to understand what fasting is, its various forms, and its historical and cultural significance. This chapter provides a comprehensive overview of fasting, setting the stage for practical application and deeper exploration in subsequent chapters.

What is Fasting?
Fasting is the voluntary abstention from food, and sometimes drink, for a specific period. Unlike starvation, fasting is a controlled practice undertaken for health, spiritual, or religious reasons. It involves deliberate intervals of eating and not eating, which can vary greatly depending on the method chosen.

Definition and History of Fasting
Fasting has been practiced for thousands of years across different cultures and religions. Historically, it has been used for spiritual purification, religious observance, and health maintenance. Ancient Greek physicians like Hippocrates recommended fasting for healing purposes, and fasting is a common practice in major religions such as Christianity, Islam, Buddhism, and Hinduism.

Different Types of Fasting

There are several types of fasting, each with its unique protocols and benefits. Understanding these variations allows individuals to choose the method that best suits their lifestyle and health goals.

Intermittent Fasting
Intermittent fasting (IF) involves cycling between periods of eating and fasting. Common IF methods include:

16/8 Method: Fasting for 16 hours and eating within an 8-hour window each day.
5:2 Diet: Eating normally for five days a week and significantly reducing calorie intake (around 500-600 calories) on two non-consecutive days.
Eat-Stop-Eat: Fasting for 24 hours once or twice a week.
Extended Fasting
Extended fasting involves fasting for more than 24 hours. Common protocols include:

48-Hour Fast: Fasting for 48 hours with no food intake.
72-Hour Fast: A three-day fast, often used to reset metabolism and jumpstart ketosis.
Water Fasting: Consuming only water for an extended period, usually 24-72 hours, or even longer under medical supervision.
Alternate-Day Fasting
Alternate-day fasting (ADF) involves alternating between days of normal eating and days of fasting or very low calorie intake (about 500 calories).

One Meal a Day (OMAD)
OMAD is a form of intermittent fasting where individuals eat one meal within a one-hour window and fast for the remaining 23 hours of the day.

Religious and Cultural Significance of Fasting

Fasting holds significant spiritual and cultural importance in many traditions:

Christianity: Lent involves 40 days of fasting or giving up certain foods or luxuries.
Islam: Ramadan is a month-long fast from dawn to sunset.
Buddhism: Monks and nuns often practice regular fasting as part of their spiritual discipline.
Hinduism: Various fasting rituals are observed, such as Ekadashi and Navratri, with specific dietary restrictions.
The Science Behind Fasting
The benefits of fasting are rooted in its impact on the body's metabolism and cellular processes.

Metabolic Changes
During fasting, the body shifts from using glucose as its primary energy source to burning fat stores. This process, known as ketosis, produces ketones, which are an efficient fuel for the body and brain.

Autophagy
Fasting triggers autophagy, a cellular cleanup process where damaged cells and proteins are recycled. This helps in cellular repair, reducing the risk of diseases like cancer and Alzheimer's.

Hormonal Changes
Fasting influences several hormones:

Insulin: Levels drop, facilitating fat burning and improving insulin sensitivity.
Human Growth Hormone (HGH): Levels increase, aiding in fat loss, muscle gain, and overall health.
Norepinephrine: Production increases, enhancing fat breakdown and providing energy.
Health Benefits of Fasting

Fasting offers numerous health benefits, including:

Weight Loss: Efficient fat burning and reduced calorie intake.
Mental Clarity: Improved focus and cognitive function due to stable blood sugar levels and increased ketones.
Longevity: Cellular repair and reduced inflammation contribute to a longer lifespan.
Blood Sugar Control: Improved insulin sensitivity and stabilized blood sugar levels.
Reduced Inflammation: Lowered markers of inflammation, reducing the risk of chronic diseases.
Enhanced Immune Function: Boosted autophagy and immune cell regeneration.
Conclusion
Understanding fasting is the first step towards harnessing its powerful benefits. By exploring the different types of fasting, their historical and cultural contexts, and the science behind them, you can make informed decisions about incorporating fasting into your lifestyle. As you continue through this book, you'll gain practical insights and strategies to help you successfully integrate fasting into your routine, ultimately transforming your health and well-being.

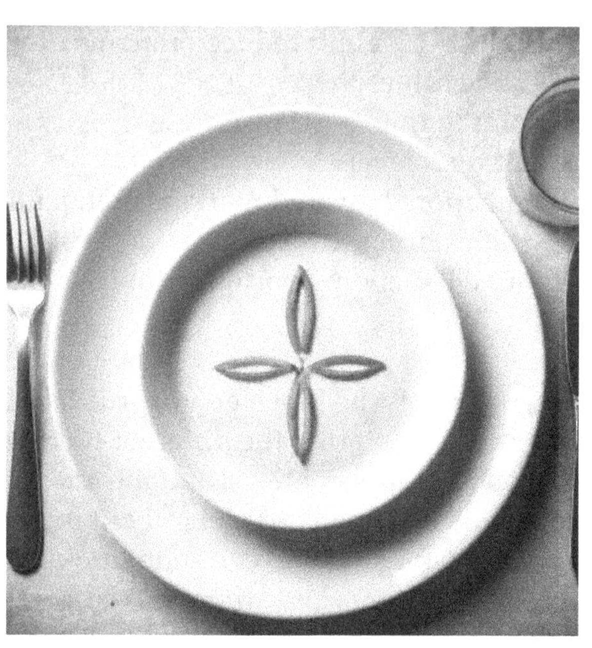

Chapter 4: What is Fasting?

Fasting is a simple yet powerful practice that involves abstaining from food and, in some cases, drink for a specified period. While the concept might seem straightforward, the nuances and variations of fasting are vast and have been utilized across different cultures and historical periods for various purposes. This chapter will define fasting, explore its historical context, and introduce different types of fasting practices.

Definition of Fasting
At its core, fasting is the voluntary abstention from food and sometimes beverages for a set period. Unlike starvation, which is involuntary and harmful, fasting is a deliberate and controlled practice often used for health, spiritual, or cultural reasons. It can range from short periods of not eating (a few hours) to extended fasting periods (several days or more).

Historical Context of Fasting
Fasting is not a new phenomenon. It has been a part of human history for thousands of years, deeply embedded in the traditions of many cultures and religions.

Ancient Practices
Ancient Greece: Fasting was recommended by ancient Greek physicians like Hippocrates, who believed in its healing properties. They used fasting to treat various ailments, promoting it as a way to cleanse the body and mind.

Early Christianity: Fasting has been a significant practice in Christianity, with early Christians observing fasting as a form of penance and spiritual discipline. Lent, a 40-day fasting period leading up to Easter, is a prominent example.

Buddhism and Hinduism: Both religions incorporate fasting into their spiritual practices. Buddhist monks often fast as part of their meditation and spiritual routine, while Hindus observe fasting during specific holy days and festivals, such as Ekadashi and Navratri.

Cultural and Religious Significance

Islam: Fasting during the month of Ramadan is one of the Five Pillars of Islam. Muslims fast from dawn to sunset, abstaining from all food and drink, to cultivate self-discipline, gratitude, and compassion for the less fortunate.

Judaism: Yom Kippur, the Day of Atonement, involves a 25-hour fast where Jews refrain from eating and drinking, focusing on prayer and repentance.

Different Types of Fasting

Understanding the various fasting methods is crucial to choosing the right one for your goals and lifestyle. Here are some of the most common types:

Intermittent Fasting (IF)

Intermittent fasting involves cycling between periods of eating and fasting. It is a flexible approach with several popular methods:

16/8 Method: This involves fasting for 16 hours each day and eating during an 8-hour window. For example, you might eat between noon and 8 PM and fast from 8 PM to noon the next day.

5:2 Diet: In this method, you eat normally for five days a week and restrict calorie intake (about 500-600 calories) on two non-consecutive days.

Eat-Stop-Eat: This involves fasting for 24 hours once or twice a week. For example, if you finish dinner at 7 PM, you wouldn't eat again until 7 PM the next day.
Extended Fasting
Extended fasting goes beyond 24 hours and can last several days. This type of fasting is more challenging and typically requires more preparation and medical supervision:

48-Hour Fast: Fasting for two days straight, consuming only water.
72-Hour Fast: A three-day fast that can help reset the body and kickstart ketosis, where the body burns fat for fuel.
Water Fasting: This involves consuming only water for the duration of the fast. It's often used for therapeutic purposes and should be done with caution and potentially under medical supervision.
Alternate-Day Fasting (ADF)
In alternate-day fasting, you alternate between days of normal eating and days where you consume very few calories (around 500-600) or none at all.

One Meal a Day (OMAD)
OMAD is a form of intermittent fasting where you eat one large meal within a one-hour window and fast for the remaining 23 hours of the day.

The Benefits and Challenges of Fasting
Each type of fasting offers unique benefits and challenges. Here's a brief overview:

Benefits: Weight loss, improved metabolic health, enhanced mental clarity, reduced inflammation, and increased longevity are among the many benefits.

Challenges: Fasting can be difficult initially due to hunger, social situations, and potential nutrient deficiencies. It requires careful planning and sometimes medical supervision, especially for extended fasts.

Conclusion

Fasting is a versatile practice with deep historical roots and a variety of methods to suit different lifestyles and health goals. Whether you're drawn to the spiritual traditions of fasting or its modern-day health benefits, understanding the different types of fasting is the first step towards incorporating this powerful practice into your life. As we continue through this book, you'll learn how to choose the right fasting method for you, prepare for your fast, and navigate the fasting process safely and effectively.

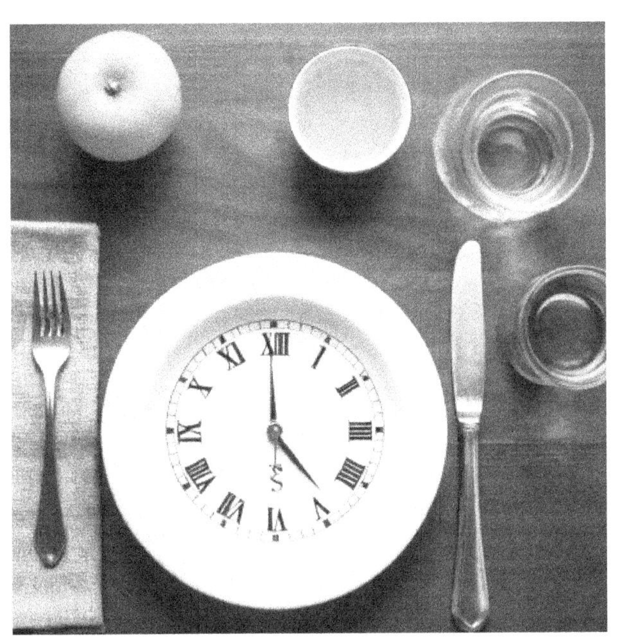

Chapter 5: Definition and History of Fasting

Fasting, the voluntary abstention from food and sometimes drink, has been practiced for millennia across various cultures and religions. Its resurgence in modern times highlights its enduring relevance and benefits. This chapter delves into the definition and history of fasting, explores its various types, and sets the stage for practical applications in later chapters.

Definition of Fasting
Fasting is the intentional avoidance of food, and occasionally drinks, for a designated period. It is different from involuntary starvation, as it is a controlled and purposeful practice often pursued for health, spiritual, or cultural reasons. The fasting periods can vary from a few hours to several days or even weeks, depending on the method and purpose.

Historical Context of Fasting
Fasting has a rich historical background, deeply embedded in the traditions and practices of numerous ancient civilizations and major religions.

Ancient Practices

Ancient Greece: Greek physicians like Hippocrates and Galen recommended fasting for its purported health benefits, such as detoxification and healing. Fasting was a common prescription for various ailments, emphasizing its therapeutic potential.

Ancient Egypt: Egyptians practiced fasting as a means of cleansing the body and preparing for spiritual rituals. It was believed to purify both the body and the soul, aligning with their holistic approach to health and spirituality.

Religious Significance

Christianity: Fasting is a significant practice in Christianity, often observed during Lent, a 40-day period of fasting and penance leading up to Easter. Early Christians used fasting as a form of spiritual discipline and penance.

Islam: Fasting during Ramadan, the ninth month of the Islamic calendar, is one of the Five Pillars of Islam. Muslims fast from dawn to sunset, refraining from all food and drink, as a means of self-discipline, spiritual reflection, and empathy for the less fortunate.

Buddhism: Buddhist monks and nuns practice fasting as part of their spiritual regimen, often abstaining from solid food after noon. Fasting is seen as a way to cultivate self-control and mindfulness.

Hinduism: Fasting is integral to Hindu practices, observed during various religious festivals like Ekadashi and Navratri. It is believed to purify the mind and body, enhancing spiritual growth.

Different Types of Fasting

Fasting can be categorized into several types, each with unique protocols and benefits. Understanding these variations helps tailor fasting practices to individual needs and goals.

Intermittent Fasting (IF)

Intermittent fasting involves cycling between periods of eating and fasting. It is flexible and can be easily integrated into different lifestyles. Common methods include:

16/8 Method: This involves fasting for 16 hours and eating within an 8-hour window each day. For example, you might eat between noon and 8 PM and fast from 8 PM to noon the next day.

5:2 Diet: In this method, you eat normally for five days a week and reduce calorie intake to about 500-600 calories on two non-consecutive days.

Eat-Stop-Eat: This involves fasting for 24 hours once or twice a week. For instance, if you finish dinner at 7 PM, you wouldn't eat again until 7 PM the next day.

Extended Fasting

Extended fasting involves abstaining from food for more than 24 hours. It is more demanding and typically requires careful preparation and sometimes medical supervision. Types include:

48-Hour Fast: Fasting for two consecutive days, consuming only water or non-caloric beverages.

72-Hour Fast: A three-day fast, which can help reset the body's metabolism and initiate deeper detoxification processes.

Water Fasting: Consuming only water for the duration of the fast, often lasting between 24-72 hours or longer under medical supervision.

Alternate-Day Fasting (ADF)

In alternate-day fasting, you alternate between days of normal eating and days where you consume very few calories (around 500-600) or none at all. This method is effective for weight loss and metabolic health improvements.

One Meal a Day (OMAD)

OMAD involves eating one large meal within a one-hour window and fasting for the remaining 23 hours of the day. This method can be challenging but is effective for those looking to simplify their eating routine and manage weight.

Benefits and Challenges of Different Fasting Types
Each fasting type offers unique benefits and challenges:

Intermittent Fasting (IF):
Benefits: Simplicity, flexibility, effective weight management, improved metabolic health.
Challenges: Initial hunger, adjusting to new eating patterns, social implications.
Extended Fasting:
Benefits: Deep detoxification, significant weight loss, enhanced autophagy.
Challenges: Physical and mental difficulty, risk of nutrient deficiencies, requires careful preparation and supervision.
Alternate-Day Fasting (ADF):
Benefits: Effective for weight loss, improves metabolic markers.
Challenges: Consistency, hunger on fasting days, potential social difficulties.
One Meal a Day (OMAD):
Benefits: Simplified eating routine, effective for weight loss and mental clarity.
Challenges: Difficulty consuming sufficient nutrients in one meal, initial hunger, social challenges.
Conclusion
Fasting is a versatile and time-honored practice with deep historical roots and a variety of modern applications. Whether through intermittent fasting, extended fasting, alternate-day fasting, or OMAD, each method offers distinct benefits and challenges. Understanding the different types of fasting allows you to choose the approach that best aligns with your health goals and lifestyle. As you continue through this book, you'll gain practical insights on how to implement fasting safely and effectively, maximizing its benefits for your overall well-being.

Chapter 6: Religious and Cultural Significance of Fasting

Fasting transcends mere dietary practice; it holds profound religious and cultural significance across the globe. This chapter explores how various religions and cultures have integrated fasting into their spiritual and communal lives, highlighting its diverse meanings and practices.

Fasting in Major Religions
Christianity
Fasting is a central practice in Christianity, symbolizing penance, purification, and spiritual discipline.

Lent: Lent is a 40-day period of fasting, reflection, and prayer leading up to Easter. Christians often give up certain foods or luxuries during this time to emulate Jesus Christ's 40-day fast in the desert.
Catholicism: Catholics observe fasting and abstinence on Ash Wednesday and Good Friday, refraining from eating meat and limiting meal portions.

Eastern Orthodox Church: The Orthodox Christian tradition includes multiple fasting periods throughout the year, including Great Lent, the Nativity Fast, and the Apostles' Fast. These fasts involve abstaining from meat, dairy, and other rich foods.

Islam

Fasting, known as Sawm, is one of the Five Pillars of Islam and is observed with great reverence.

Ramadan: During the month of Ramadan, Muslims fast from dawn to sunset, refraining from all food and drink. This fast is intended to cultivate self-discipline, spiritual growth, and empathy for the less fortunate. The fast is broken each day with a meal called Iftar, and the pre-dawn meal is called Suhoor.

Eid al-Fitr: The end of Ramadan is marked by the festival of Eid al-Fitr, a celebration of breaking the fast with communal prayers, feasts, and charitable acts.

Buddhism

Fasting in Buddhism is practiced as a means of enhancing spiritual focus and discipline.

Monastic Fasting: Buddhist monks and nuns often practice regular fasting, typically refraining from eating after noon. This practice helps to reduce attachment to food and cultivate mindfulness.

Observance Days: Lay Buddhists may fast on Uposatha days, which occur four times a month, coinciding with the lunar calendar. These days are reserved for intensified meditation, ethical observance, and spiritual reflection.

Hinduism

Fasting is deeply ingrained in Hinduism and is observed in various forms for religious and spiritual reasons.

Ekadashi: Ekadashi is observed twice a month, on the 11th day of each lunar fortnight. Devotees fast from grains and beans, and often consume only fruits and milk.

Navratri: Navratri is a nine-day festival dedicated to the goddess Durga. Many Hindus fast during this period, abstaining from certain foods and focusing on spiritual practices and rituals.

Maha Shivaratri: On Maha Shivaratri, devotees of Lord Shiva observe a strict fast, often staying awake all night and engaging in prayers and rituals.

Cultural Significance of Fasting

Ancient Cultures

Ancient Egypt: Egyptians practiced fasting for both health and spiritual purification. It was believed to prepare individuals for religious rituals and ceremonies.

Ancient Greece: Greeks used fasting as a therapeutic practice, as well as a preparatory act for spiritual and religious ceremonies. It was seen as a way to purify the body and mind.

Modern Cultural Practices

Detox Fasting: In contemporary culture, fasting is often embraced for its detoxification benefits, promoted by wellness and health movements.

Protest Movements: Fasting has been used as a form of peaceful protest. Notable examples include Mahatma Gandhi's hunger strikes for India's independence and modern-day activists using fasting to draw attention to social and political issues.

The Universal Themes of Fasting

Despite the diversity of fasting practices, several universal themes emerge:

Spiritual Discipline: Fasting is universally seen as a means of cultivating self-control, mindfulness, and spiritual discipline.

Purification: Many traditions view fasting as a way to cleanse the body and mind, preparing individuals for religious rituals and spiritual experiences.

Empathy and Compassion: Fasting often aims to develop empathy for the less fortunate, encouraging charitable acts and a deeper understanding of others' struggles.
Community and Solidarity: Fasting fosters a sense of community and solidarity, as individuals come together to observe fasts and celebrate their completion.
Conclusion
Fasting holds significant religious and cultural importance across the world. Whether practiced as a form of spiritual discipline, a means of purification, or a demonstration of empathy and solidarity, fasting transcends mere abstention from food. It is a powerful practice that connects individuals to their faith, community, and inner selves. Understanding these diverse fasting traditions enriches our appreciation of fasting's profound impact on human life. As you explore fasting in your own life, consider the deep cultural and spiritual roots that underscore this timeless practice.

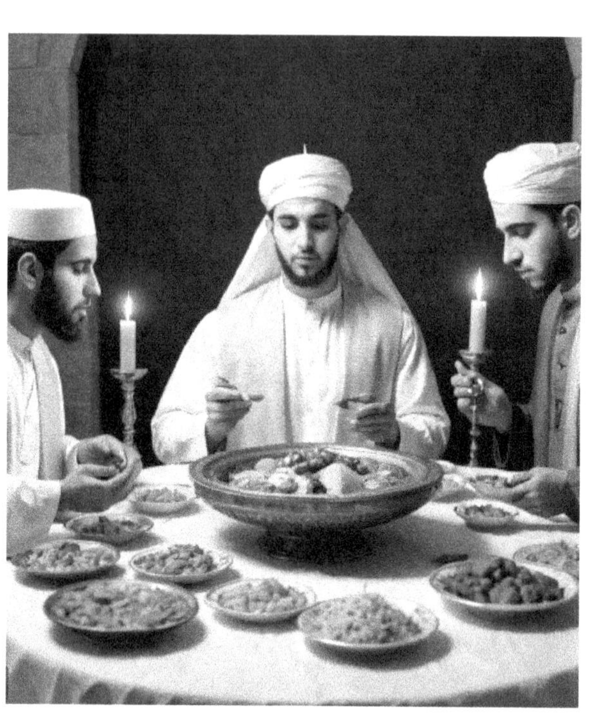

Chapter 7: The Science Behind Fasting

The resurgence of fasting in modern times is not merely due to its historical and cultural significance but is also backed by compelling scientific evidence. This chapter delves into the physiological and biochemical processes triggered by fasting, explaining how fasting affects metabolism, promotes cellular repair through autophagy, and influences hormonal changes that contribute to its myriad health benefits.

Metabolic Changes During Fasting
Fasting initiates a series of metabolic shifts as the body adapts to the absence of food intake. These changes are fundamental to understanding the benefits of fasting.

Glycogen Depletion
Initial Phase: Within the first 8-12 hours of fasting, the body utilizes glycogen stored in the liver and muscles to maintain blood glucose levels. Glycogen is a readily accessible form of glucose and serves as the primary energy source during short-term fasting.

Transition to Fat Burning: Once glycogen stores are depleted, the body shifts to burning fat for energy. This metabolic switch is crucial for sustained energy production during longer fasting periods.

Ketosis

Ketone Production: As the body breaks down fatty acids, it produces ketones, which serve as an alternative fuel source for the brain and other organs. Ketosis is a metabolic state that enhances fat burning and provides a steady supply of energy.

Benefits of Ketosis: Ketones are a more efficient fuel for the brain, leading to improved cognitive function and mental clarity. Additionally, ketosis promotes fat loss, preserves muscle mass, and stabilizes blood sugar levels.

Autophagy: Cellular Cleanup and Repair

One of the most significant benefits of fasting is the activation of autophagy, a cellular process that plays a vital role in maintaining cellular health and longevity.

What is Autophagy?

Definition: Autophagy is a process where cells degrade and recycle damaged or dysfunctional components, such as proteins and organelles. It is a critical mechanism for cellular maintenance and repair.

Mechanism: During fasting, the decrease in insulin and increase in glucagon levels trigger autophagy. The process involves the formation of autophagosomes, which engulf cellular debris and fuse with lysosomes for degradation.

Benefits of Autophagy

Cellular Health: Autophagy helps eliminate damaged cells and promotes the regeneration of healthy cells, reducing the risk of diseases like cancer and neurodegenerative disorders.

Longevity: Enhanced autophagy contributes to increased lifespan and improved overall health by maintaining cellular function and preventing the accumulation of cellular waste.

Disease Prevention: Autophagy plays a protective role against conditions such as Alzheimer's disease, Parkinson's disease, and certain cancers by removing toxic proteins and damaged cellular components.

Hormonal Changes During Fasting

Fasting induces significant hormonal changes that contribute to its health benefits. These changes help regulate metabolism, fat storage, and overall health.

Insulin

Decrease in Insulin Levels: Fasting leads to a reduction in insulin secretion, which lowers blood glucose levels and promotes fat burning.

Improved Insulin Sensitivity: Lower insulin levels enhance insulin sensitivity, reducing the risk of insulin resistance and type 2 diabetes.

Human Growth Hormone (HGH)

Increase in HGH: Fasting significantly boosts the production of human growth hormone, which plays a crucial role in muscle growth, fat metabolism, and overall health.

Benefits of HGH: Elevated HGH levels support fat loss, muscle preservation, improved physical performance, and anti-aging effects.

Norepinephrine

Fat Mobilization: Fasting increases the production of norepinephrine, a hormone that enhances fat breakdown and mobilization, providing a steady energy supply during fasting periods.

Energy and Focus: Increased norepinephrine levels contribute to improved alertness, focus, and energy levels, counteracting the potential lethargy associated with calorie restriction.

Health Benefits of Fasting

The metabolic and hormonal changes induced by fasting underpin a wide range of health benefits.

Weight Loss and Fat Loss

Caloric Deficit: Fasting naturally reduces calorie intake, leading to weight loss.

Enhanced Fat Burning: The shift to fat metabolism and ketosis promotes efficient fat loss while preserving lean muscle mass.

Improved Mental Clarity and Focus

Ketone Utilization: Ketones provide a stable and efficient energy source for the brain, enhancing cognitive function and mental clarity.

Reduced Inflammation: Fasting reduces inflammation and oxidative stress, which are linked to cognitive decline and neurological diseases.

Enhanced Longevity and Anti-Aging Effects

Cellular Repair: Autophagy promotes cellular repair and regeneration, slowing the aging process and reducing the risk of age-related diseases.

Hormonal Balance: Increased HGH levels and improved insulin sensitivity contribute to better metabolic health and longevity.

Better Blood Sugar Control and Insulin Sensitivity

Stabilized Blood Sugar Levels: Fasting helps maintain stable blood sugar levels by reducing insulin spikes and improving glucose metabolism.

Reduced Risk of Diabetes: Improved insulin sensitivity lowers the risk of developing type 2 diabetes and related metabolic disorders.

Reduced Inflammation and Improved Immune Function

Anti-Inflammatory Effects: Fasting reduces pro-inflammatory cytokines and markers of inflammation, benefiting overall health and disease prevention.

Enhanced Immune Response: Fasting boosts immune cell regeneration and function, improving the body's ability to fight infections and diseases.

Conclusion

The science behind fasting reveals its profound impact on metabolism, cellular health, and overall well-being. Through mechanisms like ketosis, autophagy, and hormonal regulation, fasting offers a powerful tool for improving health and longevity. As we continue exploring the practical aspects of fasting in the following chapters, this scientific foundation will help you understand how to harness the benefits of fasting safely and effectively.

Chapter 8: How Fasting Affects Metabolism and Cellular Processes

Fasting profoundly influences both metabolism and cellular function, orchestrating a series of biological changes that promote health and longevity. In this chapter, we will delve into how fasting affects metabolism, the critical role of autophagy, and the hormonal shifts that underpin these processes.

Fasting and Metabolism
Fasting triggers several metabolic changes as the body adapts to the absence of food. These changes are crucial for understanding the benefits of fasting.

Glycogen Depletion and Fat Burning

Glycogen Depletion: During the first 8-12 hours of fasting, the body depletes its glycogen stores in the liver and muscles to maintain blood glucose levels. Glycogen is a form of stored carbohydrate that provides a quick source of energy.

Shift to Fat Burning: Once glycogen stores are exhausted, the body transitions to burning fat for energy. This metabolic shift is a fundamental aspect of fasting, enabling prolonged periods without food intake.

Ketosis

Ketone Production: When fat is broken down, the liver produces ketones, which serve as an alternative energy source, particularly for the brain. This state of ketosis enhances fat metabolism and provides a steady energy supply.

Benefits of Ketosis: Ketones are a more efficient fuel for the brain, leading to improved mental clarity and cognitive function. Ketosis also helps stabilize blood sugar levels and supports weight loss by promoting fat burning.

The Role of Autophagy and Its Benefits

Autophagy is a critical cellular process activated by fasting, playing a vital role in maintaining cellular health and longevity.

What is Autophagy?

Definition: Autophagy, meaning "self-eating," is the process by which cells degrade and recycle damaged or dysfunctional components, such as proteins and organelles. This mechanism is essential for cellular maintenance and repair.

Mechanism: During fasting, the decrease in insulin levels and increase in glucagon levels stimulate autophagy. The process involves the formation of autophagosomes, which engulf cellular debris and fuse with lysosomes for degradation.

Benefits of Autophagy

Cellular Health: By eliminating damaged cells and promoting the regeneration of healthy cells, autophagy helps maintain cellular function and reduces the risk of diseases like cancer and neurodegenerative disorders.

Longevity: Enhanced autophagy contributes to increased lifespan and improved overall health by preventing the accumulation of cellular waste and promoting efficient cellular repair.

Disease Prevention: Autophagy plays a protective role against conditions such as Alzheimer's disease, Parkinson's disease, and certain cancers by removing toxic proteins and damaged cellular components.

Hormonal Changes During Fasting

Fasting induces significant hormonal changes that regulate metabolism, fat storage, and overall health.

Insulin

Decrease in Insulin Levels: Fasting leads to a reduction in insulin secretion, which lowers blood glucose levels and promotes fat burning.

Improved Insulin Sensitivity: Lower insulin levels enhance insulin sensitivity, reducing the risk of insulin resistance and type 2 diabetes. This improvement in insulin sensitivity is crucial for maintaining stable blood sugar levels and overall metabolic health.

Human Growth Hormone (HGH)

Increase in HGH: Fasting significantly boosts the production of human growth hormone, which is vital for muscle growth, fat metabolism, and overall health.

Benefits of HGH: Elevated HGH levels support fat loss, muscle preservation, improved physical performance, and anti-aging effects. HGH also plays a role in cellular repair and regeneration, contributing to overall health and longevity.

Norepinephrine

Fat Mobilization: Fasting increases the production of norepinephrine, a hormone that enhances fat breakdown and mobilization, providing a steady energy supply during fasting periods.

Energy and Focus: Increased norepinephrine levels contribute to improved alertness, focus, and energy levels, counteracting potential lethargy associated with calorie restriction.

Conclusion

Fasting orchestrates a complex interplay of metabolic and cellular processes that offer profound health benefits. By triggering glycogen depletion, promoting fat burning and ketosis, activating autophagy, and inducing favorable hormonal changes, fasting supports weight loss, enhances cognitive function, and improves overall health.

Understanding these scientific mechanisms provides a robust foundation for harnessing the full potential of fasting in your wellness journey. As we continue to explore the practical aspects of fasting in the upcoming chapters, this knowledge will empower you to implement fasting safely and effectively, maximizing its benefits for your health and well-being.

Chapter 9: Health Benefits of Fasting

Fasting offers a multitude of health benefits that extend beyond mere weight loss. This chapter explores two significant advantages of fasting: weight loss and fat loss, and improved mental clarity and focus. Understanding these benefits will help you appreciate the transformative potential of fasting and motivate you to incorporate it into your lifestyle.

Weight Loss and Fat Loss
One of the most compelling reasons people turn to fasting is its effectiveness in promoting weight loss and fat loss. The mechanisms through which fasting achieves these results are multifaceted and rooted in metabolic changes.

Caloric Restriction and Energy Balance
Caloric Deficit: Fasting naturally reduces overall calorie intake by limiting eating windows or entire days of food consumption. This caloric deficit is fundamental for weight loss, as it forces the body to utilize stored fat for energy.

Increased Fat Oxidation: During fasting, the body shifts from using glucose to burning fat as its primary energy source. This metabolic switch enhances fat oxidation, promoting more efficient fat loss.

Hormonal Regulation

Insulin Reduction: Fasting lowers insulin levels, a hormone that facilitates fat storage. Reduced insulin levels enhance fat burning and prevent new fat accumulation.

Increased Human Growth Hormone (HGH): Fasting boosts the production of HGH, which supports fat metabolism and preserves lean muscle mass, crucial for effective weight management.

Norepinephrine Production: Elevated levels of norepinephrine during fasting enhance fat breakdown, further promoting fat loss.

Enhanced Metabolic Rate

Short-Term Metabolic Boost: Contrary to the fear that fasting slows metabolism, short-term fasting can temporarily boost metabolic rate due to increased norepinephrine levels. This boost aids in more effective calorie burning.

Preservation of Lean Muscle Mass

Muscle Maintenance: Fasting, especially intermittent fasting, helps preserve lean muscle mass while promoting fat loss. The increased HGH levels and the body's reliance on fat for energy ensure muscle tissue is not sacrificed during fasting periods.

Improved Mental Clarity and Focus

Beyond physical benefits, fasting has a profound impact on mental health, enhancing cognitive function, mental clarity, and focus.

Ketone Utilization

Brain Fuel: During fasting, the body produces ketones as an alternative energy source. Ketones are a highly efficient fuel for the brain, providing a stable energy supply that improves cognitive function.

Neuroprotection: Ketones have neuroprotective properties, supporting brain health and protecting against cognitive decline and neurological diseases.

Reduction in Inflammation and Oxidative Stress

Anti-Inflammatory Effects: Fasting reduces markers of inflammation, which are linked to cognitive impairment and various neurological disorders. Lower inflammation levels contribute to better brain health and mental clarity.

Oxidative Stress Reduction: By decreasing oxidative stress, fasting helps protect brain cells from damage, promoting overall cognitive health.

Enhanced Neuroplasticity

Brain-Derived Neurotrophic Factor (BDNF): Fasting increases the production of BDNF, a protein that supports neurogenesis (the growth of new neurons) and enhances synaptic plasticity (the ability of synapses to strengthen or weaken over time). Higher BDNF levels are associated with improved memory, learning, and cognitive function.

Stress Resistance: The mild stress imposed by fasting stimulates adaptive responses in the brain, enhancing its resilience to stress and improving mental performance.

Improved Mood and Mental Well-Being

Endorphin Production: Fasting can increase the production of endorphins, the body's natural "feel-good" hormones, which enhance mood and overall mental well-being.

Emotional Stability: Stable blood sugar levels and improved hormonal balance during fasting contribute to better mood regulation and emotional stability.

Conclusion

The health benefits of fasting extend well beyond simple calorie restriction. By promoting weight loss and fat loss through enhanced metabolic processes and hormonal regulation, fasting offers a powerful tool for managing body weight and improving physical health. Simultaneously, fasting's impact on mental clarity and focus, driven by ketone utilization, reduced inflammation, and enhanced neuroplasticity, underscores its potential to enhance cognitive function and overall mental well-being. As you integrate fasting into your routine, these benefits can transform your health, providing a comprehensive approach to both physical and mental wellness.

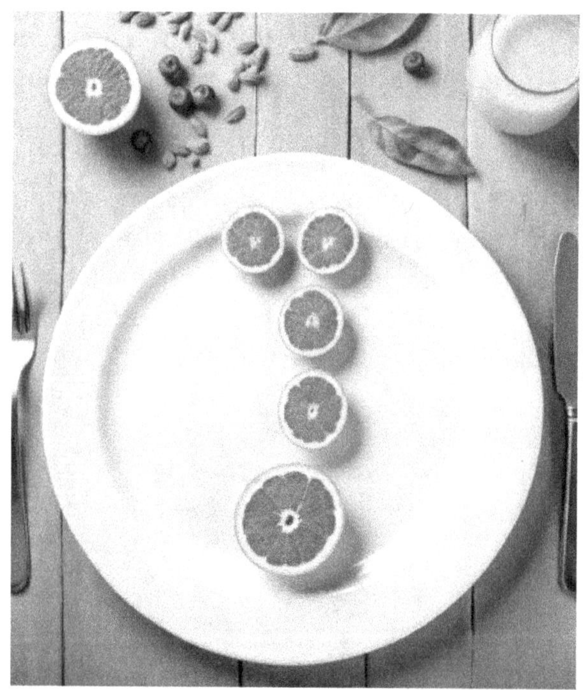

Chapter 10: Enhanced Longevity and Anti-Aging Effects

Fasting isn't just about immediate health benefits; it holds promise for extending lifespan and promoting anti-aging effects. This chapter explores how fasting contributes to longevity, enhances blood sugar control and insulin sensitivity, and reduces inflammation while boosting immune function.

Enhanced Longevity

Fasting has been linked to increased longevity through various biological mechanisms that promote cellular health and resilience.

Cellular Repair and Regeneration
Autophagy: Fasting stimulates autophagy, a process where cells break down and recycle damaged components. This cleansing mechanism rejuvenates cells and supports their longevity.
Mitochondrial Health: Fasting enhances mitochondrial function, the powerhouse of cells responsible for energy production. Improved mitochondrial health is associated with longevity and reduced cellular aging.
Hormonal Regulation
Human Growth Hormone (HGH): Fasting increases HGH production, which aids in cellular repair, regeneration, and overall metabolic health. HGH promotes tissue repair and supports a youthful physiological state.
Oxidative Stress Reduction
Antioxidant Response: Fasting triggers antioxidant pathways that counteract oxidative stress, a key contributor to aging and age-related diseases. Reduced oxidative stress supports cellular longevity and overall healthspan.
Better Blood Sugar Control and Insulin Sensitivity
Fasting plays a pivotal role in regulating blood sugar levels and improving insulin sensitivity, crucial for preventing diabetes and metabolic disorders.

Stable Blood Sugar Levels
Glucose Regulation: Fasting helps stabilize blood glucose levels by reducing insulin resistance and promoting efficient glucose metabolism. This stability is essential for overall health and disease prevention.
Insulin Sensitivity

Improved Insulin Response: Fasting lowers insulin levels and enhances insulin sensitivity, allowing cells to more effectively utilize glucose for energy. Improved insulin sensitivity reduces the risk of type 2 diabetes and promotes metabolic health.

Reduced Inflammation and Improved Immune Function

Fasting exerts anti-inflammatory effects and enhances immune function, bolstering the body's defense mechanisms against infections and diseases.

Anti-Inflammatory Response

Inflammatory Markers: Fasting reduces inflammatory markers such as cytokines and C-reactive protein (CRP), which are linked to chronic inflammation and disease. Lower inflammation levels support overall health and vitality.

Immune System Boost

Immune Cell Regeneration: Fasting promotes immune cell regeneration and enhances their function, improving the body's ability to fight infections and maintain immune balance.

Gut Health

Microbiome Balance: Fasting influences gut microbiota composition, promoting a healthy gut environment. A balanced microbiome supports immune function and reduces inflammation throughout the body.

Conclusion

Fasting offers profound benefits for longevity, anti-aging effects, blood sugar control, and immune function. By promoting cellular repair through autophagy, regulating hormones like HGH, enhancing insulin sensitivity, and reducing inflammation, fasting supports overall health and resilience. These mechanisms not only contribute to extending lifespan but also improve healthspan, the period of life spent in good health. Incorporating fasting into your lifestyle can optimize these processes, providing a powerful tool for promoting longevity, vitality, and overall well-being. As we explore practical applications of fasting in the following chapters, understanding these anti-aging and health-promoting effects will empower you to harness the full potential of fasting for a healthier and more vibrant life.

Chapter 11: Getting Started with Fasting

Embarking on a fasting journey requires preparation, understanding, and personalized planning. This chapter serves as your comprehensive guide to getting started with fasting, helping you choose the right fasting method, prepare mentally and physically, navigate through your fast, and safely break your fast.

Choosing the Right Fasting Method for You
Fasting is not one-size-fits-all; different methods suit different lifestyles and health goals. Understanding your options is crucial before beginning your fasting journey.

Overview of Popular Fasting Protocols
Intermittent Fasting (IF): Includes daily fasting windows such as 16/8 (16 hours fasting, 8 hours eating) or 18/6, where you eat within a specified time frame each day.
Extended Fasting: Involves fasting for 24 hours or more, occasionally up to several days or weeks.
Water Fasting: Abstaining from all food and drink except water for a designated period.
Alternate-Day Fasting: Alternating between fasting days and non-fasting days.
Modified Fasting: Variations that allow for limited caloric intake on fasting days, such as the 5:2 method (five days of regular eating, two days of restricted calories).
Choosing Based on Goals and Lifestyle
Weight Loss: Methods like intermittent fasting and extended fasting are effective for promoting weight loss and fat burning.

Health Maintenance: Shorter fasting windows or modified fasting methods can support overall health and metabolic function.

Spiritual or Cultural Reasons: Consider fasting periods aligned with religious or cultural practices, respecting traditional fasting guidelines.

Personalizing Your Fasting Schedule

Schedule Flexibility: Adapt fasting schedules to fit your daily routine, work schedule, and social commitments.

Gradual Adjustment: Start with shorter fasting windows and gradually increase duration as your body adapts.

Monitoring Progress: Track how different fasting methods affect your energy levels, mood, and overall well-being to find what works best for you.

Preparing for Your First Fast

Successful fasting starts with mental and physical preparation to ensure a smooth experience and maximize benefits.

Mental and Emotional Preparation

Mindset Shift: Approach fasting with a positive mindset, focusing on health benefits and personal goals.

Educate Yourself: Learn about fasting principles, benefits, and potential challenges to build confidence and reduce anxiety.

Set Realistic Expectations: Understand that fasting is an adjustment; anticipate challenges and be patient with yourself.

Physical Preparation

Nutritional Balance: Eat a balanced diet rich in whole foods before starting a fast to ensure adequate nutrient stores.

Hydration: Begin your fast well-hydrated, and maintain hydration throughout with water, herbal teas, or electrolyte supplements.

Supplement Considerations: Consult with a healthcare provider about supplements that may support fasting, such as electrolytes or vitamins.

Navigating Your Fast

During the fasting period, practical strategies can help manage hunger, maintain energy, and ensure safety.

Tips for Managing Hunger and Cravings
Stay Busy: Engage in activities that keep your mind occupied and distract from food thoughts.
Hydration: Drink water or herbal tea to curb hunger and stay hydrated.
Mild Exercise: Gentle activities like walking or yoga can help manage appetite and maintain energy levels.
Staying Hydrated and Balancing Electrolytes
Water Intake: Consume adequate water throughout the fast to prevent dehydration.
Electrolyte Balance: Supplement with electrolytes as needed to maintain balance and prevent symptoms like headaches or fatigue.
Safe Exercise Practices While Fasting
Low-Intensity Exercise: Light exercise is generally safe during fasting, but listen to your body and avoid strenuous activities.
Timing Exercise: Plan exercise sessions during periods of higher energy, such as shortly before breaking your fast.
Breaking Your Fast
How you break your fast is crucial for ensuring digestive comfort and maximizing the benefits of fasting.

Importance of Breaking Your Fast Correctly
Start Slowly: Begin with small portions of easily digestible foods to ease the digestive system back into action.
Nutrient-Dense Foods: Choose foods rich in vitamins, minerals, and proteins to replenish nutrients.
Avoid Overeating: Resist the urge to overeat after fasting; instead, listen to your body's hunger cues and eat mindfully.
Recommended Foods to Eat After Fasting
Lean Proteins: Chicken, fish, tofu, or legumes provide essential amino acids for muscle repair.

Healthy Fats: Avocado, nuts, and olive oil offer satiety and support hormone production.

Complex Carbohydrates: Whole grains and vegetables provide sustained energy and fiber for digestive health.

Refeeding Syndrome and Prevention

Gradual Transition: Avoid sudden changes in diet or large meals that can overwhelm the digestive system.

Monitor Symptoms: Be aware of signs of refeeding syndrome, such as nausea, dizziness, or electrolyte imbalances, and seek medical attention if necessary.

Conclusion

Getting started with fasting requires thoughtful consideration of your goals, lifestyle, and personal health. By choosing the right fasting method, preparing mentally and physically, navigating through your fast with practical strategies, and breaking your fast safely, you can embark on a fasting journey that supports your health and well-being. As you explore fasting further in subsequent chapters, these foundational practices will empower you to embrace fasting as a sustainable and beneficial aspect of your lifestyle.

Chapter 12: Choosing the Right Fasting Method for You

Fasting comes in various forms, each offering unique benefits and challenges. This chapter serves as a guide to understanding popular fasting protocols, such as 16/8, 5:2, OMAD (One Meal a Day), and extended fasting, helping you select the method that aligns best with your goals, lifestyle, and personal preferences.

Overview of Popular Fasting Protocols
1. 16/8 Method (Time-Restricted Eating)
Description: Involves fasting for 16 hours daily and restricting eating to an 8-hour window.
Benefits: Supports weight loss, improves metabolic health, and simplifies meal planning.
Suitability: Ideal for beginners due to flexibility and ease of integration into daily routines.
2. 5:2 Method (Modified Fasting)
Description: Involves eating normally for five days a week and restricting calorie intake to 500-600 calories on two non-consecutive fasting days.
Benefits: Promotes weight loss, enhances metabolic flexibility, and provides variety in eating patterns.
Suitability: Suited for those seeking intermittent fasting benefits with less stringent fasting periods.
3. OMAD (One Meal a Day)
Description: Restricts daily eating to a single meal within a 1-hour to 4-hour window, fasting for the remaining 20-23 hours.
Benefits: Simplifies meal planning, promotes fat loss, and may improve insulin sensitivity.

Suitability: Best for individuals comfortable with prolonged fasting periods and seeking efficient weight management solutions.

4. Extended Fasting (24+ Hours)

Description: Involves fasting for periods ranging from 24 hours to several days or even weeks.

Benefits: Enhances autophagy, promotes deep fat burning, resets insulin sensitivity, and supports mental clarity.

Suitability: Requires careful planning, hydration management, and consideration of individual health conditions.

How to Choose the Best Method Based on Individual Goals and Lifestyle

Consider Your Health Goals

Weight Loss: Methods like 16/8, 5:2, and OMAD are effective for promoting fat loss and weight management.

Metabolic Health: Intermittent fasting (16/8, 5:2) improves insulin sensitivity and supports metabolic flexibility.

Longevity and Cellular Health: Extended fasting stimulates autophagy and promotes cellular repair and regeneration.

Assess Your Lifestyle Factors

Daily Routine: Choose a fasting method that integrates seamlessly with your work, exercise, and social schedule.

Personal Preferences: Consider your food preferences, tolerance for hunger, and comfort with longer fasting durations.

Health Conditions: Consult with a healthcare provider if you have medical conditions that may affect fasting suitability.

Personalizing Your Fasting Schedule

Tailor your fasting approach to optimize adherence and maximize benefits based on individual preferences and responses.

Gradual Adjustment

Start Slowly: Begin with shorter fasting windows and gradually increase fasting duration as your body adapts.

Experiment: Test different protocols to find the one that aligns best with your energy levels, hunger cues, and overall well-being.

Flexibility: Modify fasting schedules as needed to accommodate travel, social events, or changes in daily routine.

Conclusion

Choosing the right fasting method is a personalized journey that requires consideration of health goals, lifestyle factors, and individual preferences. Whether you opt for a daily time-restricted eating window like 16/8, intermittent fasting variations such as 5:2, OMAD for simplicity, or extended fasting for deeper health benefits, understanding these protocols empowers you to harness fasting as a sustainable and effective tool for improving health and well-being. As you explore fasting further in subsequent chapters, these insights will guide you in customizing a fasting regimen that fits seamlessly into your lifestyle while delivering transformative health benefits.

Chapter 13: Preparing for Your First Fast

Embarking on your first fast requires careful preparation to ensure a smooth and successful experience. This chapter focuses on the essential aspects of mental and emotional preparation, what to eat before starting a fast, and setting realistic goals and expectations to maximize the benefits of fasting.

Mental and Emotional Preparation
Preparing mentally and emotionally is crucial for embracing fasting as a positive and transformative experience.

Understanding Fasting Benefits
Educate Yourself: Learn about the physiological benefits of fasting, such as improved insulin sensitivity, enhanced mental clarity, and weight management.
Mindset Shift: Approach fasting with a positive attitude, viewing it as a journey towards better health rather than a deprivation.
Setting Intentions
Clarify Your Goals: Define why you're fasting—whether for weight loss, metabolic health, spiritual reasons, or overall well-being. Align your intentions with your personal values.
Visualize Success: Imagine the benefits of fasting, such as increased energy, improved focus, and a sense of accomplishment.
Mental Strategies

Stay Mindful: Practice mindfulness techniques to stay present and manage cravings or hunger pangs effectively.

Build Resilience: Anticipate challenges and develop coping strategies, such as deep breathing exercises or journaling, to navigate emotional triggers during fasting.

What to Eat Before Starting a Fast

Preparing your body with the right nutrition before fasting can ease the transition and support overall well-being.

Balanced Nutrition

Whole Foods: Prioritize nutrient-dense foods such as lean proteins, whole grains, fruits, and vegetables to ensure adequate vitamins, minerals, and antioxidants.

Healthy Fats: Incorporate sources like avocados, nuts, and olive oil to promote satiety and stabilize blood sugar levels.

Hydration: Drink plenty of water and herbal teas to maintain hydration levels before fasting.

Timing of Meals

Meal Timing: Consider finishing your last meal a few hours before beginning your fast to allow for digestion and minimize discomfort.

Avoid Heavy Foods: Steer clear of heavy, processed foods, and excessive sugars that can cause digestive distress or energy crashes during fasting.

Setting Realistic Goals and Expectations

Establishing achievable goals and expectations helps maintain motivation and ensures a positive fasting experience.

Gradual Progression

Start Small: Begin with shorter fasting periods, such as 12-14 hours, and gradually increase duration based on comfort level and tolerance.

Monitor Progress: Track physical and emotional changes, such as energy levels, mood, and cravings, to gauge the effectiveness of your fasting regimen.

Health Check

Consultation: If you have pre-existing medical conditions or concerns, consult with a healthcare professional before starting your fast to ensure safety and appropriateness.

Listen to Your Body: Honor your body's signals and adjust your fasting approach accordingly to promote sustainable health benefits.

Conclusion

Preparing for your first fast involves nurturing both your mental readiness and physical readiness. By cultivating a positive mindset, fueling your body with nutrient-rich foods, and setting realistic goals, you pave the way for a successful fasting experience. As you embark on this journey towards improved health and well-being, these preparations will empower you to embrace fasting as a transformative tool for achieving your health goals and enhancing overall vitality.

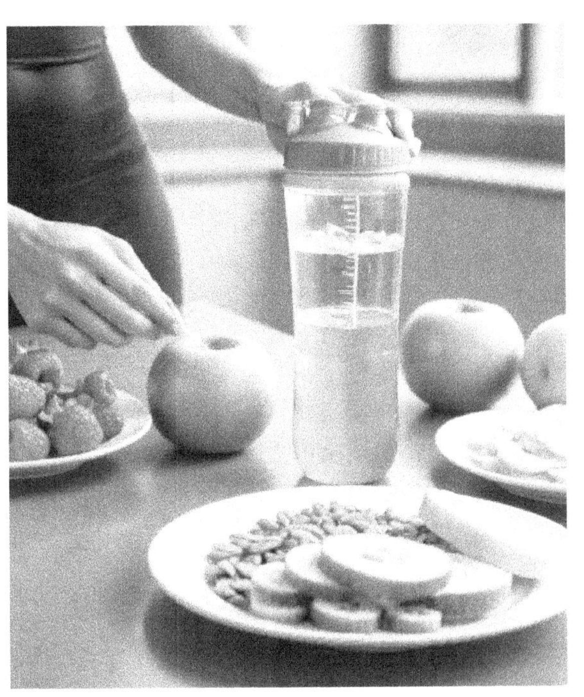

Chapter 14: Navigating Your Fast

Once you've begun your fast, navigating through it requires practical strategies to manage hunger, maintain hydration, balance electrolytes, and incorporate safe exercise practices. This chapter provides essential tips to support your fasting journey effectively.

Tips for Managing Hunger and Cravings
Managing hunger and cravings is essential to sustaining your fast and achieving its benefits.

Psychological Strategies
Stay Busy: Engage in activities such as reading, walking, or hobbies to distract yourself from thoughts of food.
Mindfulness Techniques: Practice mindfulness or meditation to observe hunger sensations without acting on them impulsively.
Progressive Relaxation: Use techniques like deep breathing or progressive muscle relaxation to reduce anxiety and manage cravings.
Practical Approaches
Stay Hydrated: Drink water, herbal teas, or infused water to help curb hunger and stay hydrated.
Consumption of Non-Caloric Beverages: Consider coffee or tea, which may also help to curb hunger.
Chew Sugar-Free Gum: This can provide a distraction and a small sense of satisfaction without breaking the fast.
Staying Hydrated and Electrolyte Balance
Maintaining hydration and electrolyte balance is crucial during fasting to support overall well-being.

Hydration Tips
Drink Water Regularly: Aim to drink at least 8-10 glasses of water per day, or more if you feel dehydrated.
Herbal Teas: Enjoy herbal teas like chamomile or peppermint for added hydration and flavor without calories.
Avoid Sugary Drinks: Steer clear of sugary beverages, which can disrupt blood sugar levels and hinder the fasting process.
Electrolyte Balance
Supplementation: Consider electrolyte supplements or drinks that provide essential minerals like sodium, potassium, and magnesium.
Natural Sources: Consume foods rich in electrolytes, such as leafy greens, nuts, seeds, and avocado, during non-fasting periods.
Safe Exercise Practices While Fasting
Incorporating exercise during fasting requires careful consideration to maintain energy levels and avoid overexertion.

Suitable Exercises
Low to Moderate Intensity: Opt for activities like walking, yoga, or gentle stretching exercises that support relaxation and promote circulation without excessive strain.
Timing: Schedule workouts during periods when you typically experience higher energy levels, such as shortly before breaking your fast or during your eating window.
Exercise Hydration
Pre-Workout Hydration: Drink water or electrolyte-rich fluids before exercise to stay hydrated and support muscle function.
Post-Workout Recovery: Rehydrate with water and consider a balanced meal to replenish nutrients and support muscle recovery after exercise.
Conclusion

Navigating through your fast involves implementing practical strategies to manage hunger, maintain hydration, balance electrolytes, and incorporate safe exercise practices. By employing these tips and techniques, you can optimize your fasting experience, support overall well-being, and maximize the health benefits of fasting. As you continue your fasting journey, adapt these practices to suit your individual needs and preferences, ensuring a sustainable and fulfilling path towards improved health and vitality.

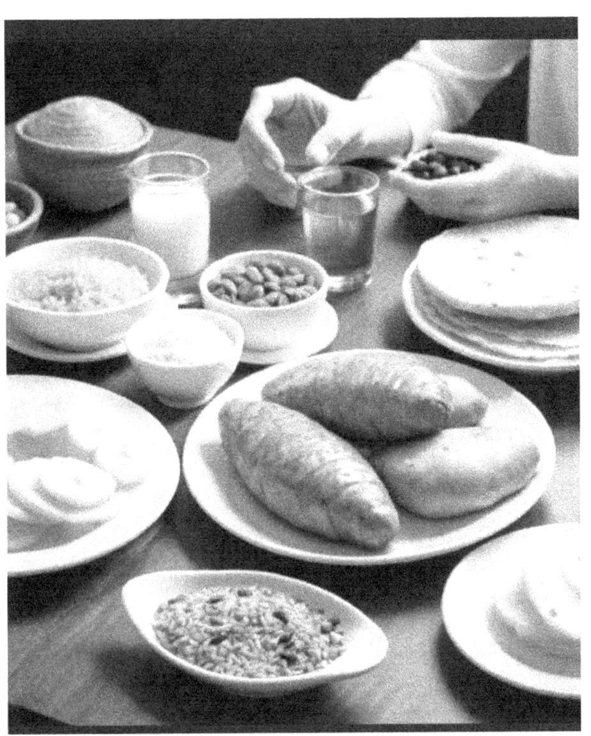

Chapter 15: Breaking Your Fast

Breaking your fast correctly is crucial for ensuring digestive comfort, replenishing nutrients, and maximizing the benefits of fasting. This chapter explores the importance of breaking your fast mindfully, recommends foods to eat after fasting, and discusses how to prevent refeeding syndrome.

Importance of Breaking Your Fast Correctly
How you end your fast sets the stage for digestion and nutrient absorption, impacting overall well-being.

Gentle Transition
Start Slowly: Begin with small portions of easily digestible foods to allow your digestive system to reawaken gradually.
Hydration: Drink water or herbal teas to hydrate your body and support digestive function.
Mindful Eating: Chew slowly and savor each bite to aid digestion and prevent discomfort.
Recommended Foods to Eat After Fasting
Choosing nutrient-dense foods promotes optimal recovery and supports metabolic health.

Nutrient-Rich Options
Lean Proteins: Chicken, fish, tofu, or legumes provide essential amino acids for muscle repair and recovery.
Healthy Fats: Avocado, nuts, seeds, and olive oil offer satiety and support hormone production.
Complex Carbohydrates: Whole grains, sweet potatoes, and vegetables provide fiber and sustained energy.
Hydration and Electrolytes
Electrolyte Balance: Consume foods rich in potassium, magnesium, and sodium to replenish electrolytes lost during fasting.

Fluid Intake: Continue to drink water and herbal teas to maintain hydration levels and support digestive processes.

Refeeding Syndrome and How to Avoid It

Refeeding syndrome can occur if nutrients are reintroduced too quickly after a prolonged fast, potentially causing serious health complications.

Understanding Refeeding Syndrome

Risk Factors: Individuals who have fasted for several days or weeks are at higher risk due to depleted electrolyte and vitamin levels.

Symptoms: Watch for signs such as nausea, dizziness, weakness, and electrolyte imbalances.

Prevention Strategies: Gradually reintroduce foods over 1-2 days, starting with small portions of easily digestible foods. Monitor symptoms closely and seek medical attention if necessary.

Conclusion

Breaking your fast mindfully and nourishing your body with nutrient-rich foods supports optimal digestion, nutrient absorption, and overall well-being. By following these guidelines for breaking your fast correctly, choosing recommended foods, and understanding how to prevent refeeding syndrome, you can enhance the benefits of fasting and promote long-term health. As you continue on your fasting journey, prioritize gradual transitions and listen to your body's signals to ensure a safe and fulfilling experience.

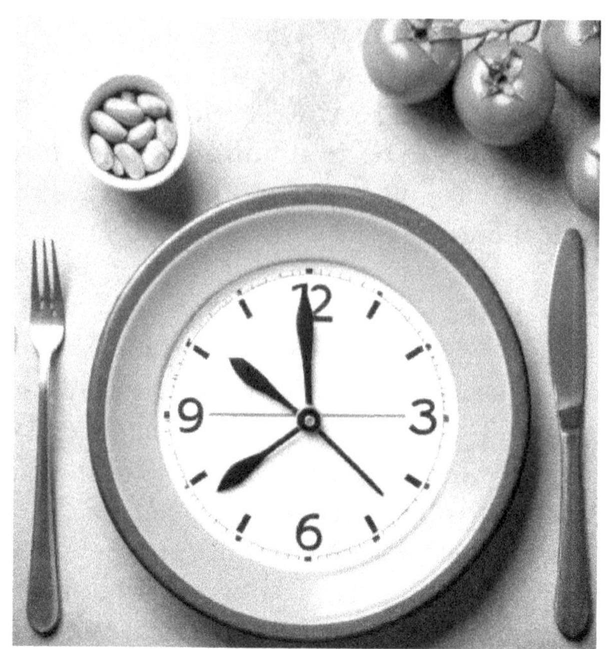

Chapter 16: Fasting for Specific Goals: Fasting for Weight Loss

Fasting has gained popularity as an effective tool for weight management, offering unique benefits that complement various dietary strategies. This chapter explores how fasting promotes weight loss, its synergies with diets like keto and low-carb, and practical tips for optimizing your fasting regimen for weight management.

How Fasting Helps with Weight Management
Fasting induces metabolic changes that facilitate fat loss and promote sustainable weight management.

Metabolic Effects
Increased Fat Burning: During fasting, insulin levels drop, prompting the body to burn stored fat for energy.
Caloric Restriction: Fasting naturally reduces calorie intake, aiding in creating a caloric deficit necessary for weight loss.
Enhanced Hormonal Balance: Fasting improves insulin sensitivity and regulates hormones like leptin and ghrelin, which influence hunger and satiety.
Sustainable Weight Loss
Long-Term Success: Fasting promotes lifestyle changes that support sustained weight loss compared to short-term diets.
Body Composition: Fasting preserves lean muscle mass while targeting fat stores, promoting a healthier body composition.
Combining Fasting with Other Dietary Strategies
Integrating fasting with complementary dietary approaches enhances metabolic flexibility and supports overall health.

Keto Diet

Synergistic Benefits: Combining fasting with a ketogenic diet enhances fat burning and promotes ketosis, a metabolic state where the body uses fat for fuel.

Improved Fat Adaptation: Fasting accelerates the transition into ketosis, maximizing the benefits of both strategies for weight loss and metabolic health.

Low-Carb Diet

Balanced Approach: Pairing fasting with a low-carb diet further stabilizes blood sugar levels and reduces insulin spikes, aiding in weight loss and managing cravings.

Enhanced Fat Loss: Low-carb diets promote fat adaptation, where the body becomes efficient at burning fat, complementing fasting's effects on metabolic efficiency.

Practical Tips for Optimizing Fasting for Weight Management

Achieving optimal results from fasting requires strategic planning and adherence to healthy practices.

Meal Planning

Nutrient-Dense Foods: Prioritize whole foods rich in vitamins, minerals, and antioxidants to support overall health and satiety.

Portion Control: Monitor portion sizes during eating windows to avoid overeating and maintain caloric balance.

Hydration and Nutrient Intake

Hydration: Drink plenty of water and electrolyte-rich fluids to support metabolism and prevent dehydration during fasting periods.

Supplements: Consider supplements like vitamins D and B12 to ensure adequate nutrient intake, especially during prolonged fasts.

Conclusion

Fasting for weight loss offers a sustainable approach to achieving and maintaining a healthy body weight. By harnessing the metabolic benefits of fasting and combining it with complementary dietary strategies such as keto or low-carb diets, individuals can optimize fat loss, improve metabolic health, and enhance overall well-being. As you explore fasting further in subsequent chapters, applying these insights will empower you to customize a fasting regimen that supports your weight management goals effectively.

Chapter 17: Success Stories and Case Studies

Real-life experiences of individuals who have embraced fasting provide compelling insights into its transformative effects. This chapter delves into success stories and case studies, illustrating how fasting has positively impacted various aspects of health and well-being.

Personal Transformation Through Fasting
Weight Loss and Body Composition
Case Study 1: Sarah's Journey to Health: Sarah struggled with obesity for years until she discovered intermittent fasting. By adopting a 16/8 fasting schedule and incorporating whole foods, she lost 50 pounds over six months, achieving her goal weight and improving her overall health.
Metabolic Health and Blood Sugar Control
Case Study 2: John's Diabetes Management: John, diagnosed with type 2 diabetes, used fasting alongside a low-carb diet to manage his condition effectively. Through intermittent fasting and regular blood sugar monitoring, he reduced his dependence on medication and improved his insulin sensitivity.
Mental Clarity and Focus
Case Study 3: Emily's Cognitive Enhancement: Emily, a professional athlete, integrated fasting with a ketogenic diet to enhance mental clarity and focus. By reducing inflammation and optimizing brain function, she experienced improved performance in competitions and daily life.
Success Stories in Longevity and Anti-Aging
Cellular Repair and Regeneration

Case Study 4: James' Anti-Aging Journey: James explored extended fasting as a means to promote cellular repair and longevity. Through periodic prolonged fasts and a nutrient-dense diet, he reported increased energy levels, reduced inflammation, and enhanced skin elasticity.

Holistic Health Improvements

Overall Well-Being and Quality of Life

Case Study 5: Maria's Holistic Wellness: Maria incorporated fasting with mindfulness practices to manage stress and improve overall well-being. By fostering a balanced lifestyle and embracing fasting as part of her routine, she achieved mental resilience and emotional well-being.

Conclusion

Success stories and case studies exemplify the diverse benefits of fasting, from weight loss and metabolic improvements to enhanced mental clarity and longevity. These narratives inspire and inform readers about the transformative potential of fasting, offering practical insights and motivation to embark on their own journey towards improved health and vitality. As you explore fasting further in subsequent chapters, these real-life examples underscore the profound impact fasting can have on individual health outcomes, empowering you to embrace fasting as a sustainable and effective tool for enhancing overall well-being.

Chapter 18: Fasting for Mental Health

Fasting not only affects physical health but also plays a significant role in enhancing mental well-being and cognitive function. This chapter explores the impact of fasting on brain health, strategies for improving focus and mental clarity, and the integration of meditation and mindfulness practices during fasting.

The Impact of Fasting on Brain Health
Cognitive Function Enhancement
Neuroplasticity: Fasting stimulates neuroplasticity, the brain's ability to adapt and reorganize, which enhances learning and memory.
Brain-Derived Neurotrophic Factor (BDNF): Fasting increases BDNF levels, promoting the growth and maintenance of neurons crucial for cognitive function.
Improved Mood: Balanced blood sugar levels and reduced inflammation from fasting can positively influence mood and emotional stability.
Strategies for Improving Focus and Mental Clarity
Cognitive Performance Optimization
Intermittent Fasting: Adopting intermittent fasting patterns, such as 16/8 or alternate-day fasting, supports sustained mental alertness and concentration.
Hydration: Maintaining adequate hydration with water and herbal teas supports brain function and reduces fatigue during fasting periods.
Healthy Fats: Incorporating healthy fats like omega-3 fatty acids from fish, nuts, and seeds can enhance cognitive function and support brain health.

Meditation and Mindfulness Practices During Fasting

Stress Reduction and Emotional Balance

Mindfulness Techniques: Practicing mindfulness meditation cultivates present-moment awareness, reducing stress and enhancing emotional resilience during fasting.

Breathing Exercises: Deep breathing exercises promote relaxation and oxygenation of the brain, enhancing mental clarity and focus.

Yoga: Gentle yoga practices improve flexibility, reduce tension, and support overall well-being during fasting.

Conclusion

Fasting offers profound benefits for mental health by enhancing brain function, improving focus, and promoting emotional balance. Integrating strategies such as intermittent fasting patterns, hydration, healthy fats, and mindfulness practices empowers individuals to optimize cognitive performance and support overall mental well-being. As you explore fasting further in subsequent chapters, these insights will guide you in harnessing fasting as a holistic approach to enhancing mental clarity, emotional resilience, and long-term brain health.

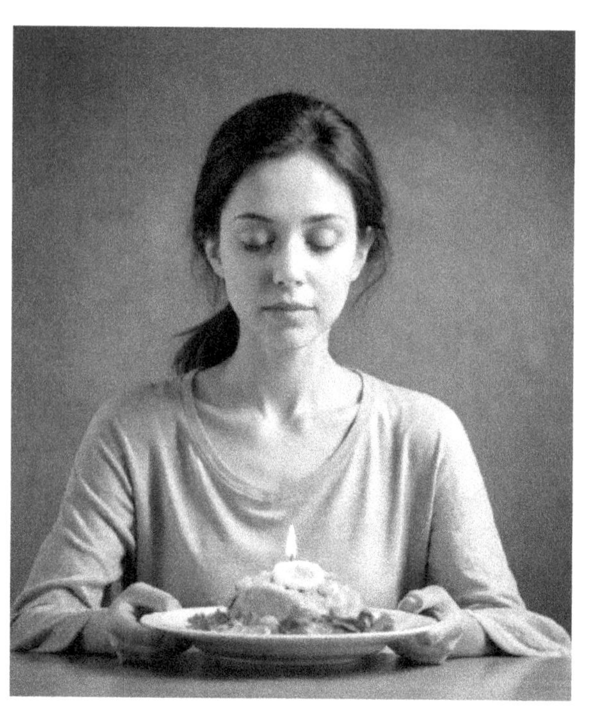

Chapter 19: Fasting for Longevity and Anti-Aging

Fasting has garnered attention not only for its weight loss benefits but also for its potential to promote longevity and slow down the aging process. This chapter explores the role of fasting in longevity, the anti-aging benefits of cellular repair and regeneration, and strategies for supplementing fasting with anti-aging nutrients.

The Role of Fasting in Promoting Longevity
Cellular Repair Mechanisms
Autophagy: Fasting triggers autophagy, a cellular process that removes damaged components and promotes renewal, contributing to longevity.
DNA Repair: Fasting may enhance DNA repair mechanisms, reducing the accumulation of DNA damage associated with aging.
Mitochondrial Health: Improved mitochondrial function through fasting supports cellular energy production and resilience against age-related decline.
Anti-Aging Benefits of Cellular Repair and Regeneration
Skin Health and Appearance
Collagen Production: Fasting may stimulate collagen synthesis, improving skin elasticity and reducing the appearance of wrinkles.
Reduced Inflammation: Lower inflammation levels from fasting contribute to skin health and overall anti-aging effects.

Gut Health: Enhanced gut microbiota balance through fasting supports nutrient absorption and reduces systemic inflammation linked to aging.

Supplementing Fasting with Anti-Aging Nutrients

Nutritional Support for Longevity

Antioxidants: Incorporate antioxidants like vitamin C, vitamin E, and polyphenols from fruits, vegetables, and green tea to combat oxidative stress and protect against cellular damage.

Omega-3 Fatty Acids: Consumption of omega-3s from fish or supplements supports brain health, cardiovascular function, and joint flexibility, contributing to overall longevity.

Resveratrol: Found in grapes and red wine, resveratrol has shown promise in promoting longevity through its antioxidant and anti-inflammatory properties.

Conclusion

Fasting offers a multifaceted approach to promoting longevity and anti-aging benefits by enhancing cellular repair mechanisms, reducing inflammation, and supporting overall health. Supplementing fasting with anti-aging nutrients such as antioxidants, omega-3 fatty acids, and resveratrol further optimizes these benefits, promoting resilience against age-related decline and supporting a vibrant, youthful lifestyle. As you delve deeper into fasting in subsequent chapters, these insights will empower you to harness its potential for longevity and anti-aging, paving the way towards a healthier and more vibrant future.

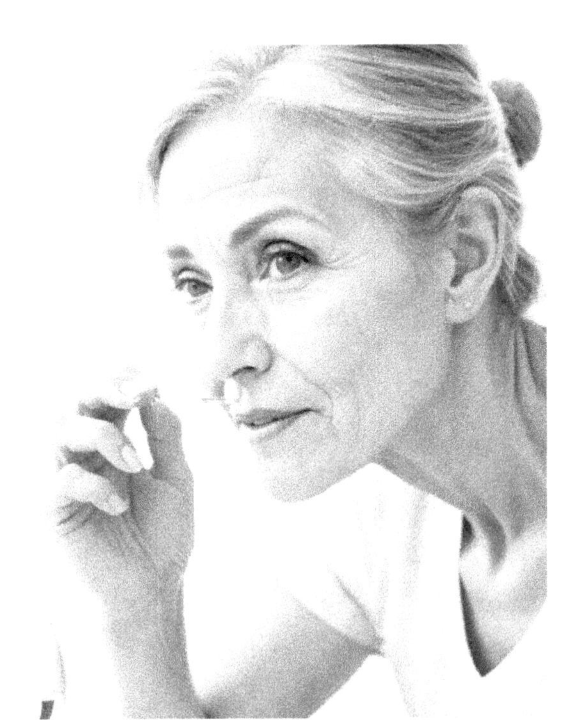

Chapter 20: Advanced Fasting Techniques: Extended Fasting Beyond 24 Hours

Extended fasting, defined as fasting periods lasting longer than 24 hours, offers profound health benefits but requires careful consideration and preparation. This chapter explores the benefits, challenges, safety considerations, and real-life experiences associated with extended fasting.

Benefits of Extended Fasting
Enhanced Cellular Repair
Autophagy: Extended fasting promotes deep autophagy, where cells repair and regenerate, removing damaged components and improving overall cellular health.
Fat Loss: Prolonged fasting accelerates fat burning as the body depletes glycogen stores and shifts to using stored fat for energy.
Insulin Sensitivity: Improved insulin sensitivity supports better blood sugar control and reduces the risk of metabolic diseases.
Challenges of Extended Fasting
Nutrient Deficiency Risk
Electrolyte Imbalance: Extended fasting may lead to electrolyte imbalances, requiring careful monitoring and supplementation.

Muscle Loss: Prolonged fasting without adequate protein intake may lead to muscle breakdown over time.

Hunger and Cravings: Managing prolonged hunger and cravings can be challenging, requiring mental resilience and strategies for distraction.

Safety Considerations and Medical Supervision

Precautions for Extended Fasting

Medical Consultation: Individuals with pre-existing medical conditions or taking medications should consult healthcare professionals before attempting extended fasting.

Monitoring Vital Signs: Regular monitoring of blood pressure, blood glucose levels, and hydration status during extended fasts is essential for safety.

Gradual Progression: Start with shorter fasting periods and gradually increase duration to acclimate the body and reduce potential risks.

Real-Life Experiences and Tips

Insights from Fasting Practitioners

Case Studies: Stories of individuals who have successfully incorporated extended fasting into their lifestyles, detailing their strategies and outcomes.

Practical Tips: Advice on managing extended fasts, including hydration, electrolyte supplementation, and mental preparation to navigate challenges effectively.

Conclusion

Extended fasting offers significant health benefits, including enhanced cellular repair, improved insulin sensitivity, and accelerated fat loss. However, it requires careful planning, safety considerations, and potentially medical supervision, particularly for prolonged fasts. By understanding the benefits, challenges, and safety precautions associated with extended fasting, individuals can explore this advanced technique safely and effectively to achieve their health and wellness goals. As you embark on your journey with fasting, incorporating these insights will empower you to navigate extended fasting with confidence and optimize its benefits for long-term health and vitality.

Chapter 21: Alternate-Day Fasting and Other Variations

Alternate-day fasting (ADF) and other variations of fasting have gained popularity for their unique approaches to health and weight management. This chapter explores alternate-day fasting, combining fasting with other diets, and experimental fasting methods, highlighting their potential benefits and considerations.

Overview of Alternate-Day Fasting (ADF)
Intermittent Caloric Restriction
ADF Patterns: Alternating between fasting days (no or minimal calorie intake) and feeding days (regular eating).

Health Benefits: ADF has shown promise in promoting weight loss, improving insulin sensitivity, and reducing inflammation.

Combining Fasting with Other Diets

Synergistic Approaches

Ketogenic Diet: Combining fasting with keto enhances fat burning and promotes ketosis, where the body uses fat for energy.

Low-Carb Diet: A low-carb diet paired with fasting stabilizes blood sugar levels and supports metabolic flexibility.

Plant-Based Diet: Fasting with a plant-based diet increases nutrient intake and promotes antioxidant and anti-inflammatory benefits.

Experimental Fasting Methods and Potential Benefits

Innovative Approaches

Time-Restricted Feeding: Narrowing the eating window (e.g., 4-hour eating window daily) improves metabolic health and supports weight management.

Fasting-Mimicking Diet: A diet that mimics fasting benefits (low calorie and high nutrient density) may offer similar health benefits without complete fasting.

Periodic Prolonged Fasting: Occasional extended fasts (e.g., 3-5 days) enhance autophagy and cellular repair, supporting longevity and metabolic health.

Practical Considerations and Implementation

Personalizing Your Approach

Health Goals: Choose a fasting method aligned with your health goals, preferences, and lifestyle.

Gradual Adaptation: Start with shorter fasting periods and gradually increase duration to acclimate your body.

Consultation: Consider consulting a healthcare professional, especially if you have medical conditions or are new to fasting.

Conclusion

Alternate-day fasting, combining fasting with other diets, and experimental fasting methods offer diverse approaches to health and wellness. By understanding the principles, benefits, and practical considerations of these fasting variations, individuals can personalize their fasting regimen to achieve optimal results. Whether exploring ADF for weight loss, combining fasting with a specific diet, or experimenting with innovative fasting methods, integrating these insights will empower you to harness fasting's potential for enhanced health, vitality, and longevity effectively. As you embark on your fasting journey, adapt and tailor these approaches to suit your individual needs, ensuring a balanced and sustainable path towards improved well-being.

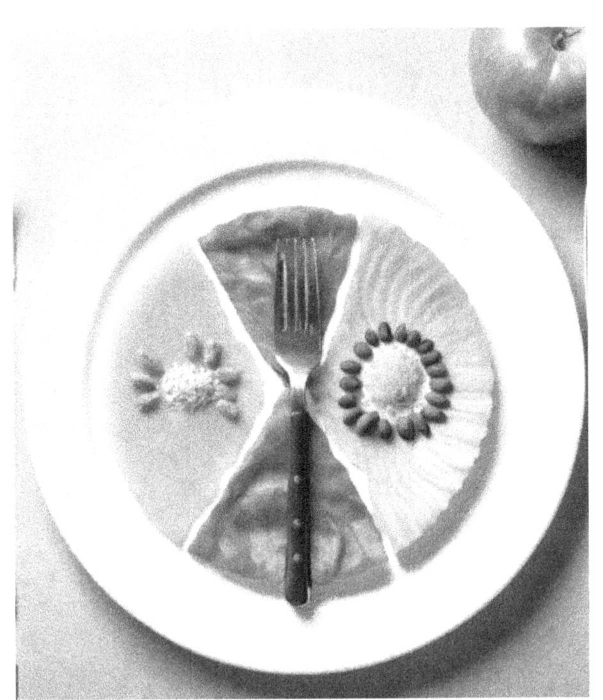

Chapter 22: Combining Fasting with Other Health Practices

Integrating fasting with various complementary health practices enhances its benefits and supports overall well-being. This chapter explores how fasting can be synergized with exercise routines, cold therapy, sauna sessions, and other biohacks, as well as holistic health practices to optimize health outcomes.

Integrating Fasting with Exercise Routines
Synergistic Benefits
Enhanced Fat Burning: Exercising in a fasted state encourages the body to burn stored fat for energy, complementing the metabolic effects of fasting.
Muscle Preservation: Fasting may preserve lean muscle mass during weight loss, especially when combined with resistance training.
Improved Endurance: Adaptation to fasting can enhance endurance performance by improving metabolic efficiency and glycogen utilization.
Synergizing Fasting with Cold Therapy, Sauna, and Other Biohacks
Metabolic and Recovery Benefits
Cold Therapy: Exposure to cold temperatures (cold showers, ice baths) enhances fat burning and metabolic rate, synergizing with fasting to promote weight loss and metabolic health.
Sauna Sessions: Heat exposure from saunas stimulates detoxification, circulation, and cardiovascular health, complementing fasting's benefits for overall well-being.

Intermittent Hypoxia: Alternating between high and low oxygen environments (hypoxic training) may enhance cellular adaptation and metabolic efficiency during fasting.

Holistic Health Practices to Complement Fasting

Mind-Body Integration

Mindfulness and Meditation: Practicing mindfulness and meditation during fasting promotes mental clarity, reduces stress, and enhances emotional resilience.

Quality Sleep: Prioritizing adequate and quality sleep supports hormone balance, cellular repair, and overall well-being during fasting.

Hydration and Nutrition: Maintaining optimal hydration and consuming nutrient-dense foods during feeding windows supports metabolic health and sustains energy levels.

Practical Tips for Integration

Personalized Approach

Gradual Implementation: Introduce new practices gradually to allow your body to adapt and maximize benefits.

Consultation: Seek guidance from healthcare professionals or trainers to tailor fasting and health practices to your individual needs and goals.

Consistency: Establishing a consistent routine with fasting and complementary practices promotes long-term adherence and optimal health outcomes.

Conclusion

Combining fasting with exercise routines, cold therapy, sauna sessions, and other biohacks offers a holistic approach to health optimization. By integrating these practices thoughtfully and consistently, individuals can enhance fat loss, improve metabolic health, and support overall well-being effectively. As you explore fasting further in subsequent chapters, applying these insights will empower you to customize a comprehensive health regimen that maximizes the benefits of fasting while promoting long-term vitality and resilience.

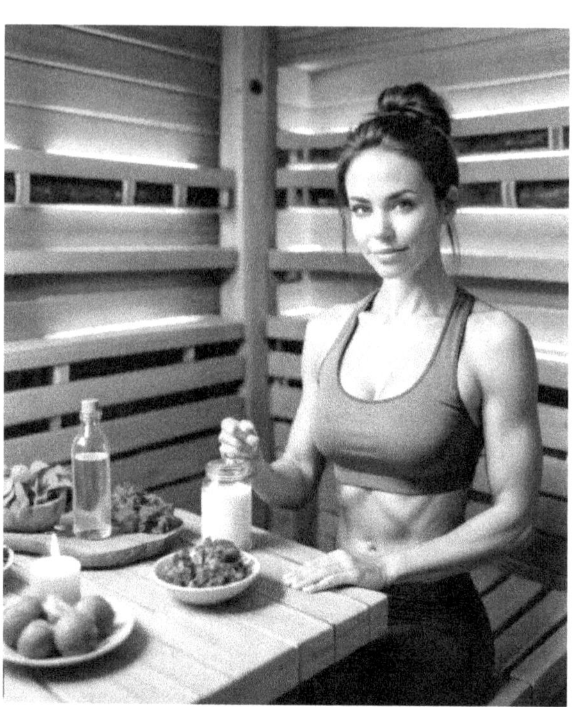

Chapter 23: Troubleshooting and Maintaining a Fasting Lifestyle

Fasting presents numerous benefits for health and well-being, yet navigating potential challenges is essential for maintaining a sustainable fasting routine. This chapter addresses common issues faced while fasting and provides practical strategies to overcome them, ensuring a successful fasting journey.

Dealing with Social Situations and Eating Out
Strategies for Social Events
Communication: Communicate your fasting schedule and dietary preferences to friends and family to manage expectations.
Flexibility: Opt for fasting-friendly options when dining out, such as salads, grilled proteins, or vegetable dishes.
Mindful Eating: Practice mindfulness to enjoy social gatherings without compromising your fasting goals.
Handling Plateaus and Adjusting Your Fasting Routine
Overcoming Plateaus
Reviewing Habits: Assess your dietary habits and fasting schedule for potential adjustments, such as varying fasting lengths or modifying meal compositions.
Physical Activity: Incorporate regular physical activity to enhance metabolism and break through weight loss plateaus.
Consultation: Seek guidance from a healthcare professional or nutritionist to personalize your fasting regimen based on your goals and health status.
Addressing Common Health Concerns

Managing Side Effects

Headaches: Stay hydrated and ensure electrolyte balance during fasting periods to alleviate headaches. Consider herbal teas or caffeine in moderation.

Fatigue: Prioritize quality sleep and nutrient-dense meals during feeding windows to combat fatigue. Incorporate relaxation techniques and manage stress effectively.

Digestive Issues: Introduce fiber-rich foods and probiotics gradually to support gut health during fasting.

Practical Tips for Long-Term Success

Sustaining a Fasting Lifestyle

Tracking Progress: Keep a journal to monitor fasting schedules, dietary intake, and health outcomes to track progress and identify patterns.

Community Support: Join online forums or local fasting groups to share experiences, gain insights, and stay motivated.

Adaptability: Embrace flexibility in your fasting routine to accommodate lifestyle changes, travel, or special occasions.

Conclusion

Troubleshooting common challenges and maintaining a fasting lifestyle requires proactive strategies and adaptability. By addressing social dynamics, overcoming plateaus, and managing health concerns effectively, individuals can sustain a balanced fasting regimen and optimize their overall health and well-being. As you continue your fasting journey, applying these practical insights will empower you to navigate challenges confidently and achieve long-term success in integrating fasting as a sustainable lifestyle choice.

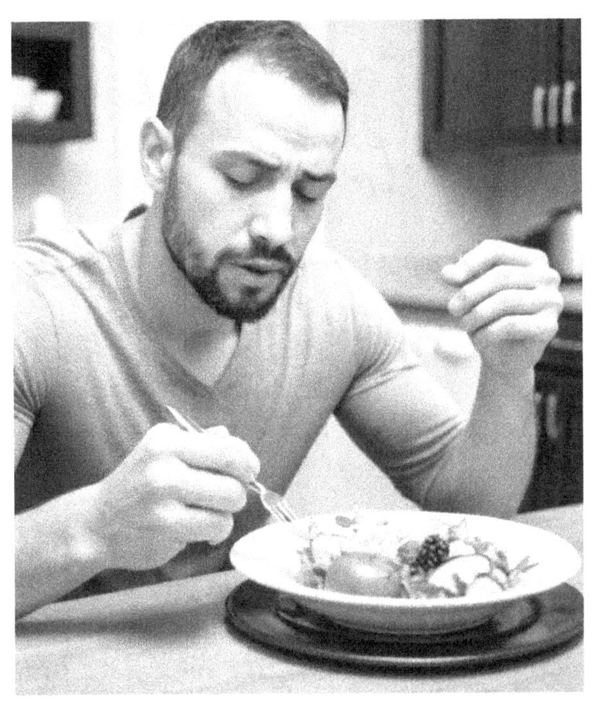

Chapter 24: Fasting Myths and Misconceptions

Fasting has gained popularity for its health benefits, yet it often faces misconceptions and criticisms. This chapter aims to debunk common myths about fasting, provide evidence-based responses to criticisms, and offer guidance on educating friends and family about the fasting lifestyle.

Debunking Common Myths About Fasting
Myth 1: Fasting Slows Down Metabolism
Reality: Short-term fasting does not slow down metabolism but can enhance metabolic flexibility and fat burning.
Evidence: Studies show fasting can increase metabolic rate during fasting periods while preserving muscle mass.
Myth 2: Fasting Leads to Muscle Loss
Reality: Properly conducted fasting, especially intermittent fasting, preserves muscle mass and promotes fat loss.
Evidence: Research indicates fasting triggers hormonal responses that protect muscle tissue and promote cellular repair.
Myth 3: Fasting Causes Nutrient Deficiencies
Reality: Fasting periods do not automatically lead to nutrient deficiencies if followed by balanced nutrition during feeding windows.
Evidence: Fasting can enhance nutrient absorption and improve insulin sensitivity, supporting overall nutrient utilization.
Evidence-Based Responses to Common Criticisms
Criticism 1: Fasting Is Unsafe or Extreme

Response: Fasting, when practiced responsibly and tailored to individual needs, can be safe and beneficial for health.

Evidence: Numerous studies support the safety and efficacy of fasting for weight management, metabolic health, and longevity.

Criticism 2: Fasting Is Not Sustainable

Response: Fasting can be sustainable when integrated into a balanced lifestyle, offering flexibility and adaptability.

Evidence: Many individuals successfully maintain fasting regimens long-term, adapting them to fit their personal preferences and schedules.

Educating Friends and Family About Your Fasting Lifestyle

Communicating Benefits and Rationale

Education: Share evidence-based benefits of fasting, such as weight loss, improved metabolic health, and enhanced cognitive function.

Personal Experience: Share your own positive experiences with fasting and how it has benefited your health and well-being.

Respect and Understanding: Acknowledge concerns and provide reassurance about safety and sustainability.

Conclusion

Understanding and addressing myths and criticisms surrounding fasting is crucial for fostering informed decisions and promoting acceptance among peers and family members. By debunking misconceptions with evidence-based responses and effectively communicating the benefits of fasting, individuals can advocate for their lifestyle choices confidently. As you navigate discussions about fasting, applying these insights will empower you to educate others positively and promote understanding of fasting as a viable and beneficial health practice.

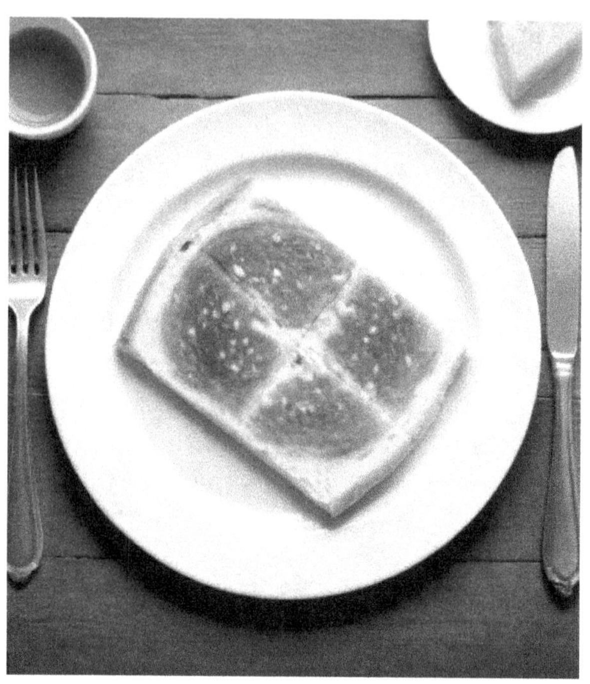

Chapter 25: Maintaining Long-Term Success

Successfully integrating fasting into your lifestyle involves creating sustainable habits, tracking progress, and staying motivated. This chapter explores strategies for establishing long-term fasting habits, monitoring your journey effectively, and maintaining motivation to achieve your health and wellness goals.

Creating Sustainable Fasting Habits
Establishing Routine and Consistency
Gradual Progression: Start with manageable fasting intervals and gradually extend them as your body adapts.
Meal Planning: Plan nutritious meals during feeding windows to support energy levels and overall well-being.
Social Support: Engage with supportive communities or partners to maintain accountability and encouragement.
Tracking Progress and Making Adjustments
Monitoring Health and Wellness
Journaling: Keep a fasting journal to record fasting schedules, dietary choices, and emotional responses.
Health Metrics: Track weight changes, body measurements, and blood markers (if applicable) to assess health improvements.
Reflection: Reflect on challenges and successes to identify patterns and make informed adjustments to your fasting routine.
Staying Motivated and Inspired
Cultivating Motivation

Setting Goals: Establish clear, realistic goals for your fasting journey, whether weight loss, improved energy, or enhanced mental clarity.

Celebrating Milestones: Celebrate achievements, no matter how small, to reinforce positive behaviors and maintain motivation.

Education and Inspiration: Stay informed about fasting benefits through books, podcasts, or seminars to stay inspired and committed.

Conclusion

Maintaining long-term success with fasting requires dedication, adaptability, and a positive mindset. By creating sustainable habits, tracking progress diligently, and staying motivated through personal goals and community support, you can maximize the benefits of fasting for improved health and well-being. As you embark on your fasting journey, apply these strategies to cultivate a balanced and fulfilling lifestyle that supports your long-term health goals effectively.

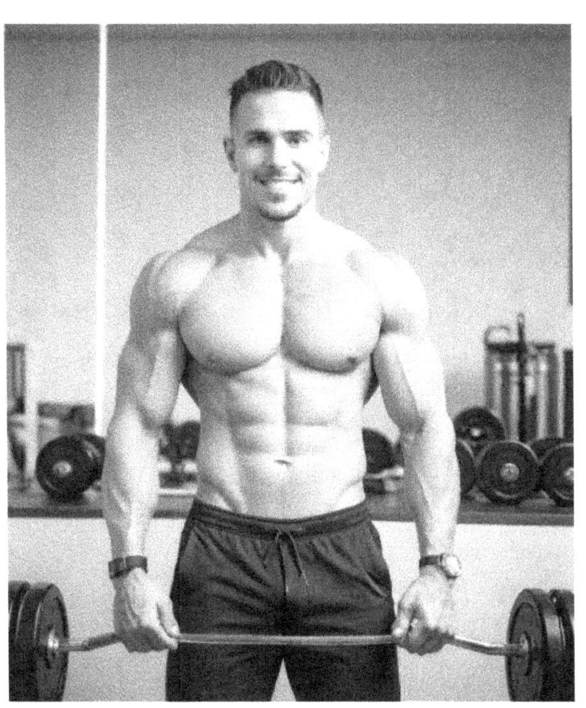

Chapter 26: Recipes and Meal Plans

Incorporating delicious and nutritious meals into your fasting routine enhances satisfaction and supports your health goals. This chapter provides a collection of pre-fasting, post-fasting, and fasting-friendly recipes, along with sample meal plans to inspire and guide your fasting journey.

Pre-Fasting and Post-Fasting Recipes
Nutrient-Rich Pre-Fasting Meals
Green Smoothie: Blend spinach, kale, avocado, and coconut water for a refreshing pre-fasting meal rich in vitamins and minerals.
Oatmeal with Berries: Cook oats with almond milk, topped with mixed berries and nuts for sustained energy before fasting.
Balanced Post-Fasting Options
Protein-Packed Salad: Combine grilled chicken, mixed greens, cherry tomatoes, cucumber, and a light vinaigrette for a satisfying post-fasting meal.
Vegetable Stir-Fry: Stir-fry broccoli, bell peppers, tofu (or lean protein of choice) with garlic and ginger for a flavorful and nutritious option.
Fasting-Friendly Recipes
Nourishing Meals During Fasting
Vegetable Broth: Simmer carrots, celery, onions, and herbs in water for a comforting and hydrating fasting-friendly broth.

Chia Seed Pudding: Mix chia seeds with almond milk and top with berries for a nutritious and filling snack during fasting periods.
Sample Meal Plans
7-Day Meal Plan for Intermittent Fasting
Day 1-5 (16/8 Method):

Breakfast: Greek yogurt with honey and walnuts
Lunch: Quinoa salad with chickpeas and mixed vegetables
Dinner: Grilled salmon with roasted sweet potatoes and steamed broccoli
Day 6 (5:2 Method):

Fast Day: Consume 500-600 calories, such as a small portion of lean protein, vegetables, and a small serving of fruit.
Day 7 (OMAD Method):

One Meal: Enjoy a balanced meal including lean protein, whole grains, and vegetables, ensuring nutritional adequacy.
Customizable Templates for Personalizing Your Meal Plan
Tailoring Meals to Your Preferences
Flexibility: Adjust portion sizes and ingredients based on dietary preferences (e.g., vegetarian, vegan) and nutritional requirements.
Variety: Explore diverse cuisines and flavors to keep meals exciting and enjoyable throughout your fasting journey.
Conclusion
Recipes and meal plans play a crucial role in supporting a successful fasting lifestyle by providing nourishing and satisfying options. Whether preparing for fasting, breaking your fast, or selecting fasting-friendly meals, these recipes and meal plans offer inspiration and guidance to maintain balanced nutrition and optimize your health journey. As you explore the culinary aspects of fasting, use these resources to create enjoyable and nutritious meals that align with your fasting goals and enhance your overall well-being.

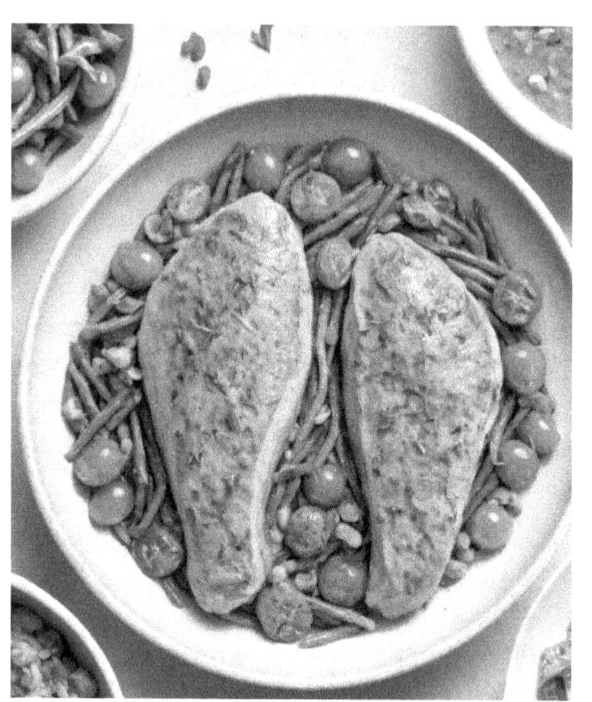

Chapter 27: Pre-Fasting and Post-Fasting Recipes

Preparing nutritious and satisfying meals before and after fasting periods is essential for maintaining energy levels and supporting overall health. This chapter offers a variety of delicious and balanced recipes tailored to enhance your fasting experience.

Pre-Fasting Recipes
Energizing and Nutrient-Dense Meals
Green Smoothie

Ingredients: Spinach, kale, avocado, banana, almond milk
Directions: Blend all ingredients until smooth. Serve chilled.
Quinoa Salad

Ingredients: Quinoa, chickpeas, cucumber, cherry tomatoes, lemon vinaigrette
Directions: Cook quinoa according to package instructions. Combine with chickpeas, cucumber, cherry tomatoes, and toss with lemon vinaigrette.
Post-Fasting Recipes
Nourishing and Balanced Options
Grilled Chicken Salad

Ingredients: Grilled chicken breast, mixed greens, bell peppers, cucumber, balsamic vinaigrette
Directions: Grill chicken until cooked through. Slice and serve over mixed greens with bell peppers and cucumber. Drizzle with balsamic vinaigrette.
Vegetable Stir-Fry

Ingredients: Broccoli, bell peppers, tofu (or protein of choice), soy sauce, garlic, ginger
Directions: Heat oil in a pan. Add garlic and ginger, followed by broccoli and bell peppers. Stir-fry until vegetables are tender. Add tofu and soy sauce. Serve hot.
Tips for Preparing and Enjoying Meals
Maximizing Nutrition and Flavor
Meal Prep: Prepare ingredients in advance to streamline meal preparation during busy periods.
Variety: Incorporate diverse fruits, vegetables, and proteins to ensure a balanced diet.
Hydration: Stay hydrated with water or herbal teas to support digestion and overall well-being.
Conclusion
These pre-fasting and post-fasting recipes provide a foundation for maintaining energy and nutrition throughout your fasting journey. By incorporating these nutritious and flavorful meals into your routine, you can optimize your fasting experience and support your health goals effectively. Whether preparing for fasting or breaking your fast, these recipes offer delicious options to enhance your overall well-being and enjoyment of the fasting lifestyle.

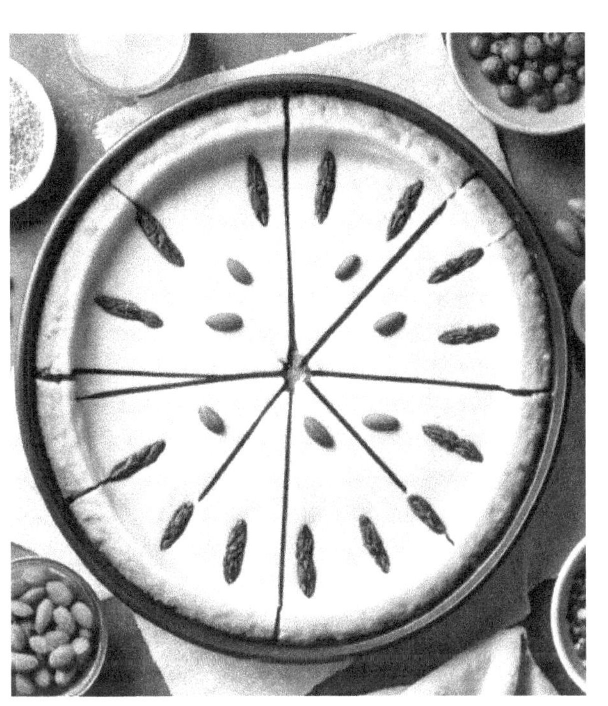

Chapter 28: Nutritious Meals Before Starting a Fast

Preparing nutritious meals before fasting is crucial to sustain energy levels and optimize nutrient intake. This chapter provides a selection of balanced and satisfying meal ideas designed to support you before embarking on a fasting period.

Balanced Meal Ideas
1. Mediterranean Quinoa Bowl
Ingredients:

Quinoa
Cherry tomatoes
Cucumber
Kalamata olives
Feta cheese
Lemon vinaigrette
Directions:

Cook quinoa according to package instructions.
Chop cherry tomatoes, cucumber, and olives.
Combine quinoa with vegetables and feta cheese.
Drizzle with lemon vinaigrette and toss gently.

2. Grilled Salmon with Sweet Potato Mash
Ingredients:

Salmon fillet
Sweet potatoes
Garlic
Olive oil
Fresh herbs (optional)
Directions:

Preheat grill or oven to cook salmon.
Peel and dice sweet potatoes, then boil until tender.
Mash sweet potatoes with garlic, olive oil, and herbs (if using).
Grill or bake salmon until cooked through.
Serve salmon with sweet potato mash.
3. Chicken and Vegetable Stir-Fry
Ingredients:

Chicken breast, sliced
Broccoli
Bell peppers
Soy sauce
Sesame oil
Ginger and garlic
Directions:

Heat sesame oil in a pan, add ginger and garlic.
Stir-fry chicken until cooked, then add broccoli and bell
peppers.
Cook until vegetables are tender-crisp.
Season with soy sauce and serve hot.
Tips for Preparation
Maximizing Nutrient Intake
Protein-Rich Choices: Include lean proteins like chicken, fish,
or tofu to support muscle maintenance.

Complex Carbohydrates: Opt for whole grains and starchy vegetables to provide sustained energy.
Fiber and Greens: Incorporate fiber-rich vegetables and leafy greens to promote digestive health.
Conclusion
These nutritious meal ideas offer a variety of options to enjoy before starting a fast, ensuring you receive essential nutrients and sustain energy levels. By selecting balanced meals rich in protein, complex carbohydrates, and vegetables, you can prepare effectively for fasting while supporting overall health and well-being. Incorporate these recipes into your routine to enhance your fasting experience and maximize the benefits of your fasting regimen.

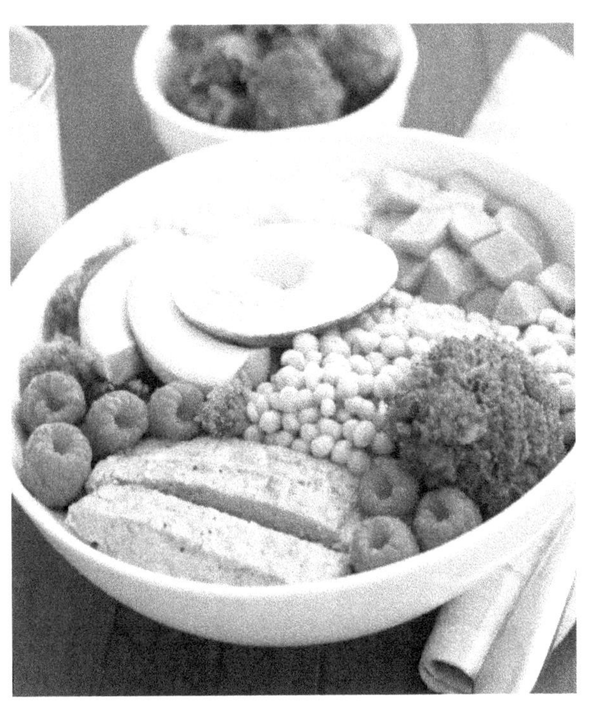

Chapter 29: Recipes for Breaking Your Fast Safely and Healthily

Breaking a fast correctly is crucial to avoid digestive discomfort and optimize nutrient absorption. This chapter presents nutritious and gentle recipes designed to reintroduce food gradually and safely after fasting periods.

Gentle and Nourishing Options
1. Vegetable Soup
Ingredients:
Assorted vegetables (carrots, celery, zucchini, spinach)
Vegetable broth
Garlic
Olive oil
Fresh herbs (parsley, thyme)
Directions:
Heat olive oil in a pot and sauté garlic until fragrant.
Add chopped vegetables and cook until slightly softened.
Pour in vegetable broth and bring to a simmer.
Cook until vegetables are tender. Season with herbs, salt, and pepper.
2. Overnight Chia Seed Pudding
Ingredients:

Chia seeds
Almond milk

Honey or maple syrup
Berries (strawberries, blueberries)
Almonds or walnuts (optional)
Directions:

Mix chia seeds with almond milk and sweetener in a bowl or jar.
Stir well and refrigerate overnight (or for at least 2 hours) until thickened.
Serve chilled with fresh berries and nuts on top.
3. Baked Sweet Potato with Avocado
Ingredients:

Sweet potatoes
Avocado
Olive oil
Sea salt
Fresh herbs (cilantro, parsley)
Directions:

Preheat oven to 400°F (200°C).
Scrub sweet potatoes and pierce several times with a fork.
Bake for 45-60 minutes until tender.
Slice open sweet potatoes, top with mashed avocado, drizzle with olive oil, and sprinkle with salt and herbs.
Tips for Breaking Your Fast Safely
Gradual Reintroduction of Foods
Start Light: Begin with easily digestible foods like soups, smoothies, or fresh fruits.
Hydration: Drink plenty of water or herbal teas to support digestion and hydration.
Listen to Your Body: Pay attention to hunger cues and proceed at a comfortable pace.
Conclusion

These recipes provide gentle and nourishing options to break your fast safely and healthily, supporting digestion and nutrient absorption. By choosing nutrient-dense foods and reintroducing them gradually, you can transition smoothly from fasting to eating, ensuring a positive and nourishing experience. Incorporate these recipes into your post-fasting routine to maintain optimal health and well-being as you continue your fasting journey.

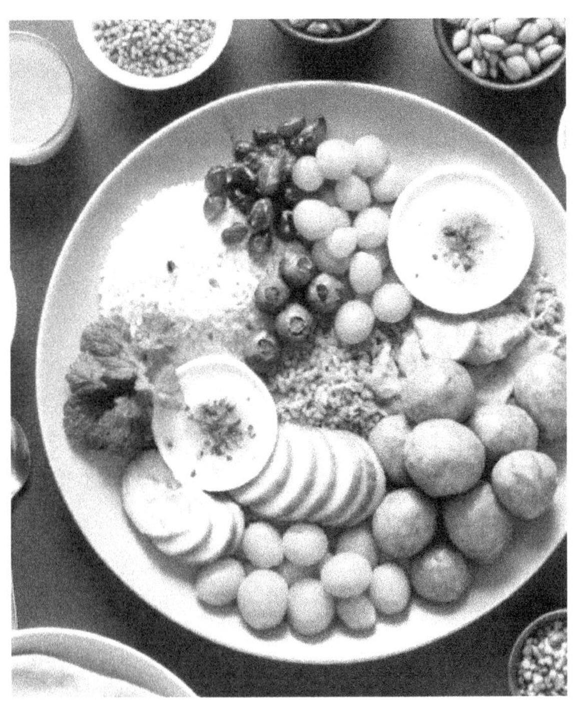

Chapter 30: Delicious and Satisfying Fasting-Friendly Recipes

Maintaining enjoyment and satisfaction during fasting periods is essential for a sustainable fasting lifestyle. This chapter offers a collection of flavorful and nourishing recipes specifically designed to support your fasting regimen.

Flavorful Fasting-Friendly Options
1. Avocado and Egg Breakfast Bowl
Ingredients:
Ripe avocado
Eggs
Cherry tomatoes
Fresh herbs (cilantro or parsley)
Salt and pepper
Directions:
Cut avocado in half and remove the pit. Scoop out some flesh to create a bowl-like shape.
Crack an egg into each avocado half.
Place avocado halves on a baking sheet and bake at 375°F (190°C) for 15-20 minutes until eggs are cooked to your liking.
Top with halved cherry tomatoes, fresh herbs, salt, and pepper.
2. Mediterranean Chickpea Salad
Ingredients:
Canned chickpeas, drained and rinsed
Cucumber, diced
Cherry tomatoes, halved
Red onion, thinly sliced

Kalamata olives, sliced
Feta cheese, crumbled
Olive oil
Lemon juice
Fresh parsley, chopped
Salt and pepper
Directions:
In a large bowl, combine chickpeas, cucumber, tomatoes, onion, olives, and feta cheese.
Drizzle with olive oil and lemon juice.
Add fresh parsley, salt, and pepper to taste. Toss gently to combine.
3. Thai-Inspired Coconut Curry Soup
Ingredients:
Coconut milk
Vegetable broth
Red curry paste
Tofu or chicken breast, cubed
Bell peppers, sliced
Bamboo shoots
Fresh basil leaves
Lime juice
Salt and pepper
Directions:
In a large pot, heat coconut milk and vegetable broth over medium heat.
Stir in red curry paste and bring to a simmer.
Add tofu or chicken, bell peppers, and bamboo shoots. Cook until protein is cooked through and vegetables are tender.
Stir in fresh basil and lime juice. Season with salt and pepper to taste.
Tips for Fasting-Friendly Cooking
Enhancing Nutritional Value
Plant-Based Proteins: Incorporate legumes, tofu, or tempeh for sustained energy and protein intake.

Herbs and Spices: Use fresh herbs and spices to enhance flavor without adding calories or disrupting fasting benefits.
Hydration: Stay hydrated with water, herbal teas, or infused water to support metabolism and curb hunger.
Conclusion
These fasting-friendly recipes offer a variety of delicious options to maintain satisfaction and nutritional balance during fasting periods. By exploring diverse flavors and incorporating nutrient-dense ingredients, you can enjoy flavorful meals that support your fasting goals and overall well-being. Incorporate these recipes into your fasting routine to enhance enjoyment and ensure sustained energy throughout your fasting journey.

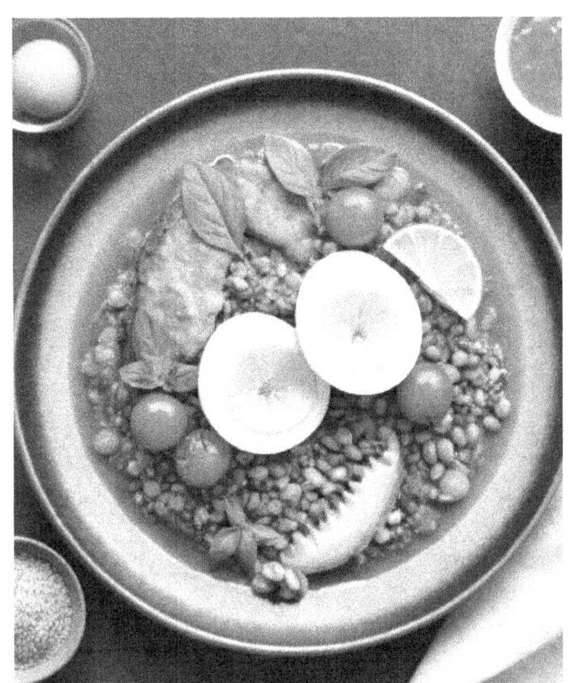

Chapter 31: Sample Meal Plans

Effective meal planning can enhance the benefits of fasting while ensuring nutritional balance and satisfaction. This chapter provides sample meal plans tailored to various fasting protocols, offering practical guidance for structuring your eating schedule and optimizing your fasting experience.

7-Day Meal Plan for Intermittent Fasting (16/8 Method)
Day 1-5:

Breakfast (12 PM): Avocado and Egg Breakfast Bowl
Lunch (3 PM): Mediterranean Chickpea Salad
Dinner (7 PM): Grilled Salmon with Sweet Potato Mash
Day 6 (Fast Day):

Hydration: Water, herbal tea, black coffee
Small Meals (500-600 Calories):
12 PM: Green Smoothie (Spinach, kale, avocado, almond milk)
3 PM: Quinoa Salad with Chickpeas
Day 7 (OMAD Method):

One Meal (6 PM): Thai-Inspired Coconut Curry Soup
Dessert: Overnight Chia Seed Pudding with Berries
5:2 Method (Two Non-Consecutive Days of Fasting)
Fast Days:

Hydration: Water, herbal tea, black coffee
Small Meals (500-600 Calories):
Breakfast: Vegetable Soup
Lunch: Baked Sweet Potato with Avocado
Feeding Days:

Day 1:

Breakfast: Avocado and Egg Breakfast Bowl
Lunch: Mediterranean Chickpea Salad
Dinner: Grilled Chicken Salad
Day 2:

Breakfast: Green Smoothie
Lunch: Quinoa Salad with Chickpeas
Dinner: Vegetable Stir-Fry with Tofu
OMAD (One Meal a Day) Method
Daily Meal (6 PM):

Meal: Thai-Inspired Coconut Curry Soup
Dessert: Overnight Chia Seed Pudding with Berries
Tips for Customizing Meal Plans
Personalization: Adjust portion sizes and ingredients based on individual calorie needs and dietary preferences (e.g., vegetarian, gluten-free).
Variety: Incorporate diverse cuisines and flavors to prevent monotony and ensure nutritional adequacy.
Hydration: Drink plenty of water throughout the day to support metabolism and curb hunger.
Conclusion
These sample meal plans offer practical examples to structure your meals according to popular fasting protocols, ensuring you achieve nutritional balance and satisfaction while optimizing the benefits of fasting. Whether you follow intermittent fasting, the 5:2 method, or OMAD, use these meal plans as a guide to support your fasting journey effectively and maintain a healthy lifestyle. Customize your meals to suit your preferences and health goals, ensuring enjoyment and success in your fasting regimen.

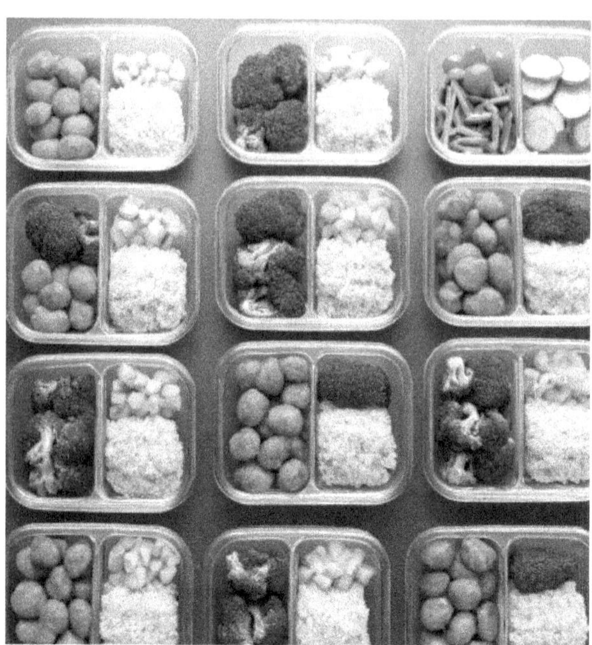

Chapter 32: 7-Day Meal Plan for Intermittent Fasting

Intermittent fasting is a popular approach that alternates between periods of eating and fasting. This 7-day meal plan provides a structured approach to intermittent fasting, focusing on nutritious meals that support energy levels and overall well-being.

Day 1
12 PM (Breakfast):

Avocado and Egg Breakfast Bowl
3 PM (Lunch):

Mediterranean Chickpea Salad
7 PM (Dinner):

Grilled Salmon with Sweet Potato Mash
Day 2
12 PM (Breakfast):

Green Smoothie (Spinach, kale, avocado, almond milk)
3 PM (Lunch):

Quinoa Salad with Chickpeas
7 PM (Dinner):

Vegetable Stir-Fry with Tofu
Day 3

12 PM (Breakfast):

Overnight Chia Seed Pudding with Berries
3 PM (Lunch):

Grilled Chicken Salad
7 PM (Dinner):

Thai-Inspired Coconut Curry Soup
Day 4 (Fast Day)
Hydration:

Water, herbal tea, black coffee
Small Meals (500-600 Calories):

12 PM: Vegetable Soup
3 PM: Baked Sweet Potato with Avocado
Day 5
12 PM (Breakfast):

Avocado Toast with Poached Egg
3 PM (Lunch):

Lentil and Vegetable Soup
7 PM (Dinner):

Baked Salmon with Roasted Vegetables
Day 6
12 PM (Breakfast):

Greek Yogurt Parfait with Berries and Almonds
3 PM (Lunch):

Spinach and Chickpea Stuffed Sweet Potato
7 PM (Dinner):

Chicken and Vegetable Stir-Fry
Day 7
12 PM (Breakfast):

Whole Grain Toast with Smashed Avocado and Tomato
3 PM (Lunch):

Quinoa and Black Bean Salad
7 PM (Dinner):

Grilled Turkey Breast with Steamed Broccoli
Tips for Success
Stay Hydrated: Drink plenty of water or herbal tea throughout the day.
Listen to Your Body: Pay attention to hunger cues and adjust meal timings as needed.
Balanced Nutrition: Incorporate a variety of proteins, vegetables, and healthy fats for optimal nutrition.
Conclusion
This 7-day meal plan offers a balanced approach to intermittent fasting, providing nourishing meals that support energy levels and overall health. Whether you're new to intermittent fasting or looking to optimize your fasting routine, use this meal plan as a guide to structure your eating schedule effectively. Customize meals based on personal preferences and nutritional needs to ensure enjoyment and success in your intermittent fasting journey.

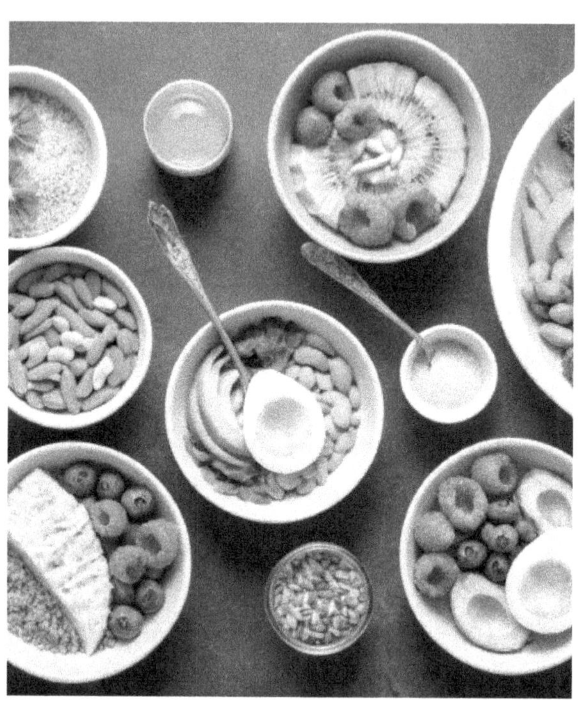

Chapter 33: Meal Plans for Various Fasting Protocols

Fasting protocols vary in their approach to alternating between eating and fasting periods. This chapter provides tailored meal plans for different fasting protocols, ensuring you can choose one that aligns with your health goals and lifestyle.

16/8 Intermittent Fasting
Eating Window: 12 PM - 8 PM

Day 1-7:

12 PM: Avocado and Egg Breakfast Bowl
3 PM: Mediterranean Chickpea Salad
7 PM: Grilled Salmon with Sweet Potato Mash
5:2 Method (Two Non-Consecutive Days of Fasting)
Fast Days (500-600 Calories):

Day 1:

12 PM: Vegetable Soup
3 PM: Baked Sweet Potato with Avocado
Feeding Days:

Day 2:

12 PM: Green Smoothie
3 PM: Quinoa Salad with Chickpeas
7 PM: Vegetable Stir-Fry with Tofu
OMAD (One Meal a Day) Method
Eating Window: 6 PM - 7 PM

Day 1-7:

6 PM: Thai-Inspired Coconut Curry Soup
Dessert: Overnight Chia Seed Pudding with Berries
Alternate-Day Fasting
Fast Days:

Day 1:

Hydration: Water, herbal tea, black coffee
Small Meals (500-600 Calories):
12 PM: Lentil Soup
3 PM: Spinach and Chickpea Stuffed Sweet Potato
Feeding Days:

Day 2:

12 PM: Avocado Toast with Poached Egg
3 PM: Quinoa and Black Bean Salad
7 PM: Grilled Turkey Breast with Steamed Broccoli
Tips for Success
Plan Ahead: Prepare meals in advance to avoid temptation during fasting periods.
Stay Hydrated: Drink water or herbal tea to stay hydrated and curb hunger.
Listen to Your Body: Adjust meal plans based on hunger levels and personal preferences.
Conclusion

These meal plans cater to various fasting protocols, offering structured approaches to optimize nutrition and support your fasting goals. Whether you choose intermittent fasting, the 5:2 method, OMAD, or alternate-day fasting, use these meal plans as a guide to maintain balance, satisfaction, and overall well-being throughout your fasting journey. Customize meals based on individual preferences and dietary needs to ensure success in achieving your health and wellness goals.

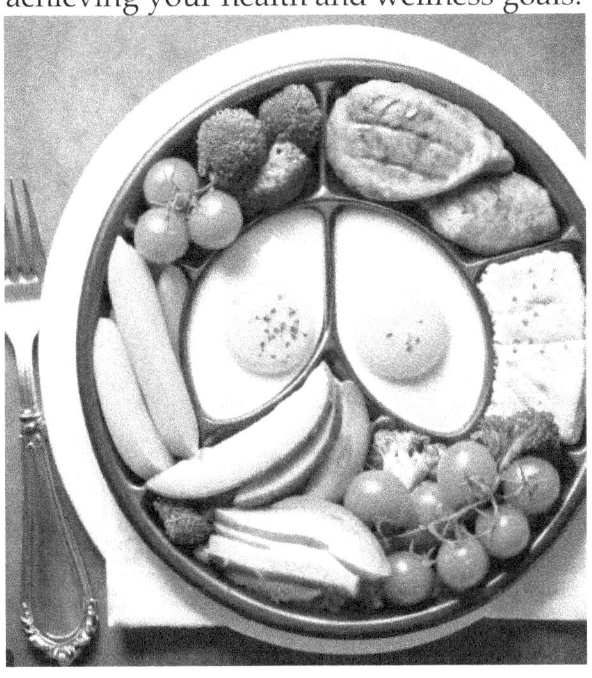

Chapter 34: Customizable Templates for Personalizing Your Meal Plan

Personalizing your meal plan is essential for adapting fasting protocols to suit your individual preferences, dietary needs, and lifestyle. This chapter provides customizable templates and guidelines to help you create a personalized meal plan that aligns with your health goals.

Template 1: Daily Intermittent Fasting Plan
Breakfast (12 PM):

Choose from: Avocado and Egg Breakfast Bowl, Green Smoothie, Greek Yogurt Parfait
Lunch (3 PM):

Choose from: Mediterranean Chickpea Salad, Quinoa Salad with Chickpeas, Lentil and Vegetable Soup
Dinner (7 PM):

Choose from: Grilled Salmon with Sweet Potato Mash, Vegetable Stir-Fry with Tofu, Baked Chicken with Roasted Vegetables
Snacks (if needed):

Choose from: Fresh fruit, nuts, yogurt with berries
Template 2: 5:2 Method Meal Plan
Fast Day (500-600 Calories):

Breakfast:

Choose from: Vegetable Soup, Green Smoothie, Chia Seed Pudding
Lunch:

Choose from: Baked Sweet Potato with Avocado, Quinoa Salad with Chickpeas, Lentil and Vegetable Soup
Feeding Day:

Breakfast (12 PM):

Choose from: Avocado Toast with Poached Egg, Greek Yogurt Parfait, Whole Grain Toast with Nut Butter
Lunch (3 PM):

Choose from: Mediterranean Chickpea Salad, Grilled Chicken Salad, Spinach and Chickpea Stuffed Sweet Potato
Dinner (7 PM):

Choose from: Thai-Inspired Coconut Curry Soup, Baked Salmon with Roasted Vegetables, Chicken and Vegetable Stir-Fry
Template 3: OMAD (One Meal a Day) Method
Meal (6 PM):

Choose from: Thai-Inspired Coconut Curry Soup, Grilled Turkey Breast with Steamed Broccoli, Quinoa and Black Bean Salad

Dessert (if desired):

Choose from: Overnight Chia Seed Pudding with Berries, Fresh Fruit with Greek Yogurt

Tips for Customizing Your Meal Plan

Caloric Needs: Adjust portion sizes and ingredients based on your daily calorie requirements.

Nutrient Balance: Include a variety of proteins, vegetables, healthy fats, and complex carbohydrates.

Dietary Preferences: Tailor recipes to accommodate vegetarian, vegan, gluten-free, or other dietary preferences.

Conclusion

Use these customizable templates as a framework to design a meal plan that meets your specific needs and supports your fasting goals effectively. By personalizing your meal plan, you can ensure enjoyment, satisfaction, and sustained progress in achieving optimal health and wellness through fasting. Experiment with different recipes, flavors, and meal timings to find the approach that works best for you and enhances your fasting experience.

Conclusion: Your Journey to a Healthier You

Congratulations on completing this comprehensive guide to fasting and its transformative impact on your health journey. Throughout this book, you've explored the profound benefits of fasting, learned about its scientific underpinnings, and discovered practical strategies to integrate fasting into your lifestyle effectively.

Reflecting on Your Progress

As you conclude this journey, take a moment to reflect on how far you've come. You've gained insights into:

Health Benefits: From weight management to enhanced mental clarity and longevity, fasting has empowered you to achieve holistic well-being.

Scientific Understanding: Understanding the metabolic and cellular processes affected by fasting has deepened your appreciation for its impact on your body.
Personal Transformation: Whether you're new to fasting or refining your approach, your dedication to personal health has laid a foundation for lasting change.
Moving Forward with Confidence

Armed with customizable meal plans, practical tips for success, and debunked myths, you're equipped to navigate challenges and maintain long-term success. Remember, your journey doesn't end here—it evolves as you continue to prioritize health and wellness.

Embracing a Healthier Lifestyle

As you embark on the next chapter of your health journey, carry forward the knowledge and empowerment gained from this book. Stay mindful of your body's needs, celebrate your achievements, and embrace the journey toward a healthier you.

Thank you for joining me on this exploration of fasting. May your path be filled with vitality, resilience, and the fulfillment of your health goals.

Here's to your continued success and well-being.

Warm regards,

Shawna Landry

Recap of Key Takeaways

Throughout this journey into the realm of fasting, several crucial insights have emerged, each contributing to a comprehensive understanding of how fasting can transform your health and well-being:

Health Benefits: Fasting offers a multitude of benefits, including weight management, improved mental clarity, enhanced longevity, and better blood sugar control.

Scientific Foundation: Delve into the science behind fasting, exploring its effects on metabolism, cellular processes like autophagy, and hormonal changes such as insulin regulation and growth hormone release.

Personalization: Choose from various fasting protocols like intermittent fasting (e.g., 16/8, 5:2), OMAD (One Meal a Day), or extended fasting, tailoring your approach to suit your lifestyle and health goals.

Preparation and Support: Prepare mentally and emotionally for fasting, set realistic goals, and seek support to navigate challenges effectively.

Nutrition and Hydration: Prioritize nutrient-dense foods and stay hydrated during fasting periods to maintain energy levels and support overall health.

Long-Term Success: Create sustainable habits, track progress, and stay motivated to ensure lasting success in your fasting journey.

Myths and Misconceptions: Address common myths surrounding fasting with evidence-based responses, educating yourself and others about its benefits.

By incorporating these key takeaways into your daily life, you can harness the power of fasting to cultivate a healthier, more vibrant you. Embrace the journey ahead with confidence, knowing that each step brings you closer to optimal health and well-being.

Encouragement and Motivation for Readers

Dear Reader,

As you conclude your exploration of fasting and embark on your personal health journey, I want to extend my heartfelt encouragement and motivation to you. Remember, embarking on a path toward better health is a courageous endeavor, and every step you take is a testament to your commitment to self-improvement and well-being.

Fasting is more than just a dietary practice—it's a transformative journey that empowers you to take control of your health and discover the incredible resilience of your body. Along the way, you may encounter challenges, both physical and emotional, but each challenge presents an opportunity for growth and learning.

Embrace the process with patience and kindness toward yourself. Celebrate your successes, no matter how small they may seem, and learn from any setbacks you encounter. Trust in your ability to adapt and thrive as you integrate fasting into your lifestyle.

Surround yourself with support—whether from loved ones, online communities, or health professionals—who can encourage you and offer guidance along the way. Share your experiences, insights, and achievements with others, fostering a community of mutual support and inspiration.

Above all, believe in the power of your choices and the potential they hold for transforming your health and quality of life. Stay committed to your goals, stay curious about your body's response to fasting, and remain open to the positive changes that lie ahead.

You have the strength and determination to achieve your health goals through fasting. Keep moving forward with confidence, knowing that each day brings you closer to a healthier, happier you.

With warmest wishes for your continued success and well-being,
Shawna

Appendices

Glossary of Terms

To aid in your understanding of fasting and its related concepts, here is a comprehensive glossary of terms used throughout this book:

Autophagy: The natural process by which the body removes and recycles damaged or dysfunctional cellular components.

Insulin: A hormone produced by the pancreas that regulates blood sugar levels and facilitates the uptake of glucose into cells for energy.

Growth Hormone: A hormone that stimulates growth, cell reproduction, and regeneration in humans and animals.

Metabolism: The set of chemical reactions that occur within the body to maintain life, including digestion, energy production, and waste elimination.

Intermittent Fasting: A pattern of eating that alternates between periods of fasting (not eating) and eating within a designated time window.

Extended Fasting: Fasting periods that extend beyond 24 hours, typically lasting several days.

Water Fasting: A type of fasting that involves consuming only water and no other food or beverages.

OMAD (One Meal a Day): A form of intermittent fasting where individuals eat one large meal within a one-hour time frame each day.

Refeeding Syndrome: A potentially serious condition that can occur when someone who is malnourished or has been fasting undergoes rapid refeeding, causing shifts in electrolytes and fluids.

Ketosis: A metabolic state in which the body uses fat for fuel instead of carbohydrates, typically achieved through a low-carbohydrate or ketogenic diet.

Caloric Restriction: A dietary regimen that reduces calorie intake without malnutrition, often associated with longevity and health benefits.

Electrolytes: Minerals in the body that carry an electric charge and regulate bodily functions, including hydration, nerve function, and muscle contraction.

This glossary is designed to enhance your comprehension and provide clarity on key terms related to fasting and its physiological effects. Refer to it as needed throughout your journey toward better health and well-being.

Frequently Asked Questions

What is intermittent fasting, and how does it work?
Intermittent fasting involves cycling between periods of eating and fasting. Common methods include the 16/8 method (16 hours of fasting with an 8-hour eating window) and the 5:2 method (eating normally for 5 days and restricting calories on 2 non-consecutive days).

What are the health benefits of fasting?
Fasting has been associated with benefits such as weight loss, improved metabolic health, enhanced mental clarity, better blood sugar control, and reduced inflammation.

Is fasting safe for everyone?

While fasting can be safe for many people, it may not be suitable for those with certain medical conditions, pregnant or breastfeeding women, or individuals with a history of eating disorders. Consult with a healthcare professional before starting a fasting regimen.

How do I choose the right fasting method for me?
Consider your lifestyle, health goals, and preferences when selecting a fasting method. Start with shorter fasting periods and gradually increase duration if desired. Experiment to find what works best for your body and schedule.

What should I eat before starting a fast?
Opt for balanced meals containing protein, healthy fats, and complex carbohydrates to sustain you during the fasting period. Avoid heavy or sugary foods that may cause energy crashes.

How can I manage hunger and cravings while fasting?
Stay hydrated with water, herbal tea, or black coffee. Incorporate fiber-rich foods and protein to promote satiety. Practice mindfulness and distraction techniques to curb cravings.

What is refeeding syndrome, and how can it be prevented?
Refeeding syndrome is a rare but potentially serious condition that can occur when someone who is malnourished or has been fasting undergoes rapid refeeding, leading to electrolyte imbalances. Gradually reintroduce foods and monitor electrolyte levels under medical supervision to prevent this.

Can fasting help with weight loss?
Fasting can aid weight loss by promoting calorie restriction and enhancing fat burning. Combined with a balanced diet and regular exercise, fasting may support sustainable weight management.

Are there risks associated with fasting?
Risks may include dehydration, electrolyte imbalances, and potential adverse effects in certain medical conditions. Always approach fasting with caution, especially if you have underlying health concerns, and seek guidance from a healthcare provider.

How can I maintain long-term success with fasting?
Establish sustainable habits, monitor progress, and adjust your fasting regimen as needed. Incorporate nutrient-dense foods and stay mindful of overall health and well-being beyond fasting.

These frequently asked questions provide essential insights into fasting, addressing common concerns and considerations to support your journey toward improved health and vitality. For personalized guidance, consult with a healthcare professional or nutrition expert.

Resources for Further Reading and Support

Expand your knowledge and find support for your fasting journey with these recommended resources, including websites, books, and forums:

Websites:
The Fasting Method - Offers comprehensive guides, articles, and resources on various fasting protocols.

Diet Doctor - Provides evidence-based information and recipes for intermittent fasting and low-carb diets.

PubMed - Access research articles and studies on fasting and its effects on health and metabolism.

Healthline - Features articles and expert advice on intermittent fasting, health benefits, and practical tips.

Books:
"The Complete Guide to Fasting: Heal Your Body Through Intermittent, Alternate-Day, and Extended Fasting" by Dr. Jason Fung and Jimmy Moore - Explores different fasting methods, their benefits, and practical advice for implementation.

"Delay, Don't Deny: Living an Intermittent Fasting Lifestyle" by Gin Stephens - Offers personal insights, success stories, and tips for integrating intermittent fasting into daily life.

"The Obesity Code: Unlocking the Secrets of Weight Loss" by Dr. Jason Fung - Discusses the role of insulin resistance and the benefits of intermittent fasting in managing weight and improving metabolic health.

Forums and Communities:
Reddit - r/intermittentfasting - Engage with a community of fasting enthusiasts, share experiences, and seek advice on various fasting methods.

Facebook Groups - Intermittent Fasting Success Stories - Connect with individuals who have experienced success with intermittent fasting, share tips, and support each other on your journey.

Online Forums - The Fast Diet Forums - Participate in discussions about intermittent fasting, share recipes, and find motivation from community members.

Additional Resources:
Podcasts - Listen to podcasts such as "The Intermittent Fasting Podcast" and "FoundMyFitness" by Dr. Rhonda Patrick for in-depth discussions on fasting and health.

Nutritionists and Healthcare Providers - Consult with a registered dietitian or healthcare professional for personalized guidance and support tailored to your health needs.

These resources offer valuable information, support, and community interaction to enhance your understanding of fasting and optimize your health journey. Explore them to find inspiration, motivation, and practical tools for achieving your wellness goals through fasting.

References and Scientific Studies Cited in the Book

For those interested in exploring the scientific foundation and evidence supporting the principles discussed in this book, here are some of the key references and scientific studies cited:

Fasting and Metabolism:

Cahill Jr GF. Fuel metabolism in starvation. Annu Rev Nutr. 2006;26:1-22.
Longo VD, Mattson MP. Fasting: molecular mechanisms and clinical applications. Cell Metab. 2014 Feb 4;19(2):181-92.
Autophagy and Cellular Processes:

Mizushima N, Komatsu M. Autophagy: renovation of cells and tissues. Cell. 2011;147(4):728-41.

Rubinsztein DC, Codogno P, Levine B. Autophagy modulation as a potential therapeutic target for diverse diseases. Nat Rev Drug Discov. 2012;11(9):709-30.

Hormonal Changes During Fasting:

Hartman ML, Veldhuis JD, Johnson ML, et al. Augmented growth hormone (GH) secretory burst frequency and amplitude mediate enhanced GH secretion during a two-day fast in normal men. J Clin Endocrinol Metab. 1992;74(4):757-65.

Anson RM, Guo Z, de Cabo R, et al. Intermittent fasting dissociates beneficial effects of dietary restriction on glucose metabolism and neuronal resistance to injury from calorie intake. Proc Natl Acad Sci U S A. 2003;100(10):6216-20.

Health Benefits of Fasting:

Patterson RE, Laughlin GA, LaCroix AZ, et al. Intermittent fasting and human metabolic health. J Acad Nutr Diet. 2015;115(8):1203-12.

Anton SD, Moehl K, Donahoo WT, et al. Flipping the metabolic switch: understanding and applying the health benefits of fasting. Obesity (Silver Spring). 2018;26(2):254-68.

Fasting for Weight Loss:

Varady KA, Bhutani S, Church EC, Klempel MC. Short-term modified alternate-day fasting: a novel dietary strategy for weight loss and cardioprotection in obese adults. Am J Clin Nutr. 2009;90(5):1138-43.

Harvie MN, Pegington M, Mattson MP, et al. The effects of intermittent or continuous energy restriction on weight loss and metabolic disease risk markers: a randomized trial in young overweight women. Int J Obes (Lond). 2011;35(5):714-27.

Fasting for Mental Health:

Fond G, Macgregor A, Leboyer M, Michalsen A. Fasting in mood disorders: neurobiology and effectiveness. A review of the literature. Psychiatry Res. 2013;209(3):253-8.
Solianik R, Sujeta A. The effect of prolonged fasting on mental performance. Med Sci Monit. 2016;22:4301-11.
Fasting for Longevity and Anti-Aging:

Fontana L, Partridge L, Longo VD. Extending healthy life span—from yeast to humans. Science. 2010;328(5976):321-6.
Lee C, Longo VD. Fasting vs dietary restriction in cellular protection and cancer treatment: from model organisms to patients. Oncogene. 2011;30(30):3305-16.
These references provide a basis for the principles discussed in the book and offer further reading for those interested in exploring the scientific aspects of fasting. Each study contributes to understanding how fasting affects metabolism, health outcomes, and longevity.

Bonus Chapter: Weight Control

Weight control, often synonymous with weight management, is the practice of maintaining a healthy body weight within a desired range for optimal health and well-being. It encompasses both preventing weight gain and, when necessary, actively working to lose weight. As an expert in the field, I can explain weight control from several perspectives:

Caloric Balance: At its core, weight control revolves around the concept of caloric balance — balancing the number of calories consumed through food and beverages with the number of calories expended through physical activity and metabolic processes. When caloric intake exceeds expenditure, weight gain occurs; when caloric intake is less than expenditure, weight loss occurs.

Factors Influencing Weight: Weight control is influenced by a complex interplay of genetic, metabolic, environmental, and behavioral factors:

Genetics: Genetic predispositions can influence metabolism, fat storage, and appetite regulation, affecting an individual's susceptibility to weight gain or obesity.
Metabolism: Basal metabolic rate (BMR) and metabolic efficiency impact how efficiently the body uses calories for energy.
Environment: Access to healthy foods, socioeconomic factors, cultural norms, and environmental cues can influence dietary choices and physical activity levels.
Behavior: Eating habits, physical activity patterns, stress management, and sleep hygiene all play significant roles in weight control.
Health Implications: Maintaining a healthy body weight is crucial for overall health and reduces the risk of chronic diseases such as type 2 diabetes, cardiovascular disease, hypertension, and certain cancers. Weight control also improves mobility, energy levels, and psychological well-being.

Strategies for Weight Control: Effective weight control strategies typically include:

Balanced Diet: Emphasizing whole foods, lean proteins, fruits, vegetables, and healthy fats while moderating intake of processed foods, sugary beverages, and high-calorie snacks.

Regular Physical Activity: Incorporating aerobic exercise, strength training, and flexibility exercises to increase calorie expenditure, improve metabolic rate, and maintain muscle mass.

Behavioral Changes: Adopting mindful eating practices, portion control, stress management techniques, and adequate sleep habits to support healthy weight management.

Medical Intervention: In cases of severe obesity or metabolic disorders, medical interventions such as medication or bariatric surgery may be considered under medical supervision.

Lifestyle Approach: Successful weight control is often best achieved through a holistic lifestyle approach that integrates dietary modifications, regular physical activity, behavior change, and ongoing self-monitoring. This approach promotes sustainable habits that support long-term weight maintenance and overall health improvement.

Personalization and Support: Recognizing that individual responses to weight control strategies vary, personalized approaches tailored to individual preferences, cultural backgrounds, and health conditions are crucial. Supportive environments, including healthcare professionals, registered dietitians, and community resources, can provide guidance, motivation, and accountability in achieving weight control goals.

Overall, weight control is a dynamic and multifaceted endeavor that requires a comprehensive understanding of individual factors, behaviors, and environmental influences to achieve and maintain a healthy body weight.

Bonus Chapter: Diet

Definition of Diet: A diet refers to the habitual eating patterns and choices of individuals or populations. It includes all foods and beverages consumed regularly, reflecting cultural, social, economic, and personal preferences.

Nutritional Components: Diets consist of macronutrients (carbohydrates, proteins, fats) and micronutrients (vitamins, minerals) essential for growth, development, and overall health. Each nutrient plays specific roles in bodily functions, from providing energy to supporting immune function and tissue repair.

Types of Diets:

Balanced Diet: Emphasizes a variety of foods from all food groups, including fruits, vegetables, whole grains, lean proteins, and healthy fats, to ensure adequate nutrient intake.
Specialty Diets: Tailored to specific health needs or preferences, such as vegetarian, vegan, gluten-free, or low-carb diets, which may require careful planning to meet nutritional requirements.
Therapeutic Diets: Prescribed to manage medical conditions like diabetes, hypertension, or allergies, focusing on controlling blood sugar levels, reducing sodium intake, or eliminating allergens.
Health Impact: A well-balanced diet is crucial for maintaining optimal health and preventing chronic diseases. Benefits include:

Weight Management: Controlling caloric intake and nutrient balance supports healthy weight maintenance or weight loss.
Disease Prevention: Nutrient-rich diets reduce the risk of cardiovascular diseases, type 2 diabetes, certain cancers, and osteoporosis.
Energy and Vitality: Proper nutrition enhances energy levels, cognitive function, and overall well-being.
Immune Function: Nutrients like vitamins A, C, D, and zinc support immune response, reducing susceptibility to infections.
Components of a Healthy Diet:

Fruits and Vegetables: Rich sources of vitamins, minerals, fiber, and antioxidants essential for cellular function and disease prevention.
Whole Grains: Provide complex carbohydrates for sustained energy, fiber for digestive health, and B vitamins for metabolism.

Proteins: Found in lean meats, poultry, fish, beans, nuts, and seeds, proteins are vital for muscle repair, immune function, and hormone production.

Healthy Fats: Unsaturated fats from olive oil, avocados, nuts, and fatty fish support heart health, brain function, and nutrient absorption.

Hydration: Water is essential for cellular hydration, temperature regulation, and nutrient transport throughout the body.

Factors Influencing Dietary Choices:

Cultural and Social Factors: Influence food preferences, cooking methods, and eating habits.

Psychological Factors: Emotions, stress, and food cravings affect food choices and eating behaviors.

Environmental Factors: Availability, accessibility, and affordability of nutritious foods impact dietary patterns.

Individual Preferences and Beliefs: Personal taste preferences, dietary restrictions, ethical considerations, and health goals shape dietary choices.

Guidelines for Healthy Eating:

Moderation: Balance portion sizes and food choices to meet nutritional needs without excessive calorie intake.

Variety: Include a diverse range of foods to ensure intake of different nutrients and phytochemicals.

Quality: Choose nutrient-dense foods over processed or high-sugar foods to optimize health benefits.

Individualization: Customize dietary plans to meet personal health goals, preferences, and lifestyle factors.

In summary, a well-planned diet is essential for promoting overall health, preventing disease, and supporting optimal physical and mental function. By understanding the principles of nutrition and making informed dietary choices, individuals can achieve and maintain a balanced and health-promoting diet tailored to their unique needs and circumstances.

Bonus Chapter: Nutrition

Definition of Nutrition: Nutrition refers to the science of how the body obtains and utilizes nutrients from food to support growth, repair, energy production, and overall health. It encompasses the study of macronutrients (carbohydrates, proteins, fats) and micronutrients (vitamins, minerals) essential for physiological functions.

Key Nutrients:

Macronutrients: Provide energy (calories) and include: Carbohydrates: Primary energy source, found in grains, fruits, vegetables.

Proteins: Essential for tissue repair, enzyme production, found in meats, dairy, legumes.
Fats: Source of energy, insulation, cell membrane structure, found in oils, nuts, avocados.
Micronutrients: Essential for metabolism, immune function, and various physiological processes:
Vitamins: Organic compounds (e.g., vitamin C, B vitamins) critical for enzyme function and metabolism.
Minerals: Inorganic elements (e.g., calcium, iron) necessary for bone health, oxygen transport, and nerve function.
Functions of Nutrients:

Energy Production: Carbohydrates, fats, and proteins are metabolized to provide ATP (adenosine triphosphate), the body's energy currency.
Tissue Repair and Growth: Proteins are essential for building and repairing tissues, including muscles, organs, and immune cells.
Metabolism: Vitamins and minerals act as cofactors for enzymatic reactions involved in metabolism, converting food into energy and synthesizing molecules.
Immune Function: Nutrients like vitamins A, C, D, and minerals such as zinc and selenium support immune response and reduce susceptibility to infections.
Cellular Function: Fatty acids and phospholipids derived from fats are integral to cell membrane structure and function.
Sources of Nutrients:

Plant-Based: Fruits, vegetables, legumes, whole grains provide fiber, vitamins, minerals, and phytochemicals.
Animal-Based: Meats, fish, dairy products supply high-quality proteins, B vitamins (especially B12), and minerals like calcium and iron.
Fats: Found in oils, nuts, seeds, and fatty fish provide essential fatty acids (omega-3 and omega-6) crucial for brain function and inflammation regulation.

Processed Foods: Often fortified with vitamins and minerals, but may also contain excessive sugars, salts, and unhealthy fats.
Nutritional Requirements:

Daily Values: Recommended dietary allowances (RDAs) and daily values (DVs) provide guidelines for nutrient intake based on age, sex, health status, and life stage.
Individual Variability: Nutritional needs vary based on factors like age, sex, metabolism, activity level, and health conditions.
Special Populations: Specific dietary needs for children, pregnant or lactating women, athletes, and older adults require tailored nutrition plans.
Impact of Nutrition on Health:

Chronic Disease Prevention: A balanced diet rich in fruits, vegetables, and whole grains reduces the risk of chronic diseases such as cardiovascular disease, diabetes, and certain cancers.
Weight Management: Proper nutrition supports healthy weight maintenance or loss by balancing caloric intake with energy expenditure.
Mental and Emotional Well-Being: Nutrients like omega 3 fatty acids, B vitamins, and antioxidants support brain function, mood regulation, and cognitive health.
Nutrition Education and Guidance:

Nutritionists and Dietitians: Provide evidence-based guidance on meal planning, dietary modifications, and nutritional counseling tailored to individual needs.
Public Health Initiatives: Promote nutrition education, healthy eating habits, and policies to improve food accessibility, quality, and safety.

In conclusion, nutrition plays a vital role in maintaining optimal health and well-being throughout life. By understanding the principles of nutrition and making informed dietary choices, individuals can support their physical, mental, and emotional health, reducing the risk of disease and promoting longevity.

Bonus Chapter: Healthy eating

Balanced Nutrition: Healthy eating involves consuming a variety of foods from all food groups in appropriate proportions to meet nutritional needs. This includes:

Fruits and Vegetables: Rich sources of vitamins, minerals, fiber, and antioxidants essential for immune function, digestion, and disease prevention.
Whole Grains: Provide complex carbohydrates, fiber, and B vitamins for sustained energy, digestive health, and metabolic function.
Proteins: Found in lean meats, poultry, fish, legumes, nuts, and seeds, proteins are crucial for muscle repair, hormone production, and enzyme function.

Healthy Fats: Unsaturated fats from sources like olive oil, avocados, nuts, and fatty fish support heart health, brain function, and nutrient absorption.

Dairy or Alternatives: Calcium-rich foods or fortified alternatives support bone health and provide essential nutrients like vitamin D and potassium.

Portion Control: Maintaining appropriate portion sizes helps manage calorie intake and prevents overeating, supporting weight management and overall health. Portion control involves being mindful of serving sizes and using visual cues or portion guidelines to avoid excessive calorie consumption.

Moderation and Variety: Healthy eating emphasizes moderation in consuming foods high in added sugars, unhealthy fats, and sodium. Variety ensures a diverse intake of nutrients and phytochemicals, reducing the risk of nutrient deficiencies and promoting overall health benefits.

Nutrient Density: Choosing nutrient-dense foods ensures optimal nutrient intake relative to calorie content. Nutrient-dense foods provide essential vitamins, minerals, and other beneficial compounds without excessive calories, supporting health and vitality.

Hydration: Adequate hydration is essential for cellular function, temperature regulation, nutrient transport, and waste elimination. Water is the primary recommendation for hydration, with additional fluids obtained from herbal teas, infused waters, and fruits.

Mindful Eating: Practicing mindful eating involves paying attention to hunger and fullness cues, savoring flavors and textures, and avoiding distractions during meals. Mindful eating promotes a healthier relationship with food, enhances digestion, and supports better food choices.

Benefits of Healthy Eating:

Disease Prevention: A well-balanced diet rich in fruits, vegetables, whole grains, and lean proteins reduces the risk of chronic diseases such as cardiovascular disease, type 2 diabetes, hypertension, and certain cancers.
Weight Management: Healthy eating habits promote sustainable weight loss or maintenance by providing essential nutrients, controlling portion sizes, and reducing the consumption of empty calories.
Energy and Vitality: Proper nutrition supports energy levels, cognitive function, and overall well-being, improving productivity and daily functioning.
Longevity and Quality of Life: Healthy eating habits contribute to longevity and enhance quality of life by reducing the impact of age-related diseases and supporting physical and mental health.
Lifestyle Approach: Healthy eating is part of a holistic lifestyle that includes regular physical activity, stress management, adequate sleep, and other health-promoting behaviors. Integrating these factors supports comprehensive well-being and sustainable health outcomes.

In summary, healthy eating involves making informed choices that prioritize nutrient-dense foods, moderation, and balance. By adopting healthy eating habits, individuals can enhance their overall health, prevent chronic diseases, and improve their quality of life.

Bonus Chapter: Healthy lifestyle

Physical Activity: Regular exercise and physical activity are foundational to a healthy lifestyle. This includes:

Aerobic Exercise: Activities like walking, jogging, swimming, or cycling that increase heart rate and improve cardiovascular health.
Strength Training: Exercises using weights or resistance bands to build muscle strength, improve bone density, and enhance metabolism.
Flexibility and Balance: Stretching exercises and activities like yoga or tai chi to maintain flexibility, posture, and reduce the risk of injuries.
Nutritious Diet: A balanced and varied diet rich in whole foods, including:

Fruits and Vegetables: Provide vitamins, minerals, fiber, and antioxidants essential for immune function and disease prevention.

Whole Grains: Complex carbohydrates for sustained energy, fiber for digestive health, and B vitamins for metabolism.

Lean Proteins: From sources like poultry, fish, beans, nuts, and seeds to support muscle repair, hormone production, and overall cellular function.

Healthy Fats: Unsaturated fats from olive oil, avocados, and fatty fish to support heart health, brain function, and nutrient absorption.

Hydration: Drinking an adequate amount of water and fluids to maintain hydration, regulate body temperature, and support bodily functions.

Stress Management: Techniques to reduce stress levels and promote mental well-being, such as:

Mindfulness and Meditation: Practices to enhance awareness, reduce anxiety, and improve emotional resilience.

Breathing Exercises: Techniques to calm the mind, lower blood pressure, and promote relaxation.

Time Management: Strategies to prioritize tasks, delegate responsibilities, and maintain a healthy work-life balance.

Adequate Sleep: Getting sufficient and quality sleep is crucial for:

Restoration and Repair: Allows the body to repair tissues, consolidate memories, and regulate hormones.

Cognitive Function: Enhances concentration, decision-making, and overall mental performance.

Mood and Emotional Well-Being: Supports emotional resilience, reduces irritability, and enhances overall mood stability.

Social Connections: Building and maintaining supportive relationships with family, friends, and community members:

Emotional Support: Provides a sense of belonging, reduces feelings of isolation, and improves overall mental health.
Social Engagement: Participating in social activities, hobbies, or group events fosters a sense of purpose and fulfillment.
Avoidance of Harmful Substances: Limiting or avoiding substances that can negatively impact health:

Tobacco: Quitting smoking or avoiding exposure to secondhand smoke to reduce the risk of lung cancer, respiratory diseases, and cardiovascular conditions.
Alcohol: Moderating alcohol consumption to minimize the risk of liver disease, hypertension, and mental health disorders.
Illicit Drugs: Avoiding illegal substances that can lead to addiction, health complications, and social consequences.
Regular Health Screenings: Proactively scheduling and attending routine medical check-ups, screenings, and vaccinations to detect and prevent health conditions early.

Continuous Learning and Personal Growth: Engaging in activities that stimulate mental agility, creativity, and lifelong learning:

Reading: Expanding knowledge, staying informed, and enhancing critical thinking skills.
Hobbies: Pursuing interests and passions that provide enjoyment, relaxation, and a sense of accomplishment.
Environmental Awareness: Making choices that promote environmental sustainability and health, such as:

Sustainable Practices: Conserving natural resources, reducing waste, and choosing eco-friendly products.
Outdoor Activities: Spending time in nature, benefiting physical and mental health through fresh air, sunlight, and exercise.

Positive Outlook and Resilience: Cultivating a positive mindset, practicing gratitude, and developing resilience to cope with challenges and setbacks effectively.

In summary, a healthy lifestyle involves integrating physical activity, nutritious eating, stress management, adequate sleep, social connections, and other positive habits into daily routines. By prioritizing these aspects, individuals can enhance their overall well-being, prevent chronic diseases, and improve their quality of life.

Bonus Chapter: Fitness

Definition of Fitness: Fitness refers to the ability to perform physical activities efficiently and effectively, encompassing several components:

Cardiorespiratory Endurance: The ability of the heart, lungs, and blood vessels to deliver oxygen to working muscles during prolonged physical activity. Improving cardiorespiratory endurance enhances stamina and reduces the risk of cardiovascular diseases.

Muscular Strength: The amount of force a muscle or group of muscles can exert against resistance in one maximal effort. Strength training exercises, such as weightlifting or bodyweight exercises, increase muscle mass, bone density, and metabolic rate.

Muscular Endurance: The ability of muscles to sustain repeated contractions against resistance without fatigue. Endurance training, such as circuit training or high-repetition weightlifting, enhances muscle stamina and improves overall fitness performance.

Flexibility: The range of motion at a joint or series of joints. Flexibility exercises, such as stretching or yoga, improve muscle elasticity, joint mobility, and posture, reducing the risk of injuries and enhancing athletic performance.

Body Composition: The proportion of fat, muscle, and bone in the body. Achieving a healthy body composition through balanced nutrition and regular exercise supports overall fitness and reduces the risk of obesity-related diseases.

Benefits of Fitness:

Physical Health: Regular exercise and physical activity improve cardiovascular health, strengthen muscles and bones, enhance flexibility and balance, and support weight management.

Mental and Emotional Well-Being: Fitness activities release endorphins, neurotransmitters that promote feelings of happiness and reduce stress, anxiety, and depression. Physical activity also improves cognitive function and enhances mental clarity.

Longevity: Maintaining a high level of fitness reduces the risk of chronic diseases, such as heart disease, diabetes, and certain cancers, leading to a longer and healthier life.

Quality of Life: Improved fitness levels enhance daily functioning, increase energy levels, and promote independence in activities of daily living, contributing to a higher quality of life as individuals age.

Components of a Fitness Program:

Cardiovascular Exercise: Activities that elevate heart rate and increase breathing rate, such as walking, running, cycling, swimming, or dancing. Aim for at least 150 minutes of moderate-intensity cardio or 75 minutes of vigorous-intensity cardio per week.

Strength Training: Exercises targeting major muscle groups using weights, resistance bands, or body weight. Include exercises for all major muscle groups at least twice a week, focusing on proper form and progression.

Flexibility and Stretching: Stretching exercises to improve flexibility and range of motion, reducing the risk of injuries and enhancing muscle elasticity. Perform static stretches after workouts or incorporate yoga or Pilates into your routine.

Balance and Stability: Exercises to improve core strength, balance, and coordination, reducing the risk of falls and enhancing overall functional fitness. Include balance exercises, such as standing on one leg or using stability balls.

Fitness Training Principles:

Progressive Overload: Gradually increasing the intensity, duration, or frequency of exercise to continually challenge the body and promote fitness gains.

Specificity: Tailoring exercise programs to meet specific fitness goals, whether improving endurance, strength, flexibility, or sports performance.

Rest and Recovery: Allowing adequate rest between workouts and ensuring proper nutrition to repair muscles, prevent overtraining, and optimize fitness gains.

Individualization: Designing fitness programs based on individual fitness levels, health status, age, and personal goals to ensure safety and effectiveness.

Getting Started with Fitness:

Consultation: Before starting a new fitness program, consult with a healthcare provider, especially if you have any pre-existing health conditions or concerns.

Goal Setting: Establish specific, measurable fitness goals (e.g., weight loss, muscle gain, improved endurance) to guide your exercise program and track progress.

Gradual Progression: Start with low-intensity exercises and gradually increase intensity, duration, and frequency to avoid injury and build stamina.

Enjoyment: Choose activities you enjoy and vary your routine to maintain motivation and prevent boredom.

In conclusion, fitness encompasses various physical components and is integral to overall health and well-being. By incorporating cardiovascular exercise, strength training, flexibility, and balance activities into a regular fitness program, individuals can enhance their physical fitness, improve mental and emotional well-being, and enjoy a higher quality of life.

Bonus Chapter: Exercise

Definition of Exercise: Exercise refers to physical activity that is planned, structured, and repetitive, with the specific purpose of improving or maintaining physical fitness. It involves the systematic engagement of muscles and joints to promote health, fitness, and overall well-being.

Types of Exercise:

Aerobic Exercise: Also known as cardiovascular or endurance exercise, aerobic activities increase heart rate and breathing for sustained periods. Examples include jogging, swimming, cycling, and dancing. Aerobic exercise improves cardiovascular fitness, increases stamina, and supports weight management.

Strength Training: Also referred to as resistance or weight training, strength exercises involve working against resistance to build muscle strength, power, and endurance. Activities include weightlifting, resistance band exercises, and bodyweight exercises like push-ups and squats. Strength training enhances muscle tone, increases metabolism, and improves bone density.

Flexibility and Stretching: Flexibility exercises aim to improve the range of motion of muscles and joints. Stretching routines, yoga, and Pilates help maintain or increase flexibility, reduce muscle stiffness, and prevent injuries.

Balance and Stability: Balance exercises enhance stability and coordination, reducing the risk of falls and injuries. Activities such as standing on one leg, using balance boards, or practicing Tai Chi improve posture and overall body control.

Functional Training: Exercises that mimic everyday movements to improve strength and endurance for daily activities. Functional training focuses on movements like bending, lifting, and reaching, promoting better mobility and reducing the risk of injury.

Benefits of Exercise:

Physical Health: Regular exercise improves cardiovascular health by strengthening the heart and improving circulation. It lowers blood pressure, reduces the risk of heart disease, stroke, and diabetes, and improves cholesterol levels.

Weight Management: Physical activity burns calories and helps maintain a healthy weight by increasing metabolism and reducing body fat. Combining aerobic exercise with strength training supports muscle growth and boosts calorie burning.

Muscle and Bone Health: Strength training exercises build muscle mass and increase bone density, reducing the risk of osteoporosis and fractures. Exercise also promotes joint health by lubricating and strengthening the supporting structures.

Mental and Emotional Well-Being: Exercise releases endorphins, neurotransmitters that promote feelings of happiness and reduce stress, anxiety, and depression. Physical activity improves mood, enhances cognitive function, and supports better sleep quality.

Longevity: Regular physical activity is associated with a longer lifespan and reduced risk of premature death from chronic diseases.

Quality of Life: Exercise enhances overall well-being by increasing energy levels, improving self-esteem, and promoting a sense of accomplishment and satisfaction.

Exercise Guidelines:

Frequency: Aim for at least 150 minutes of moderate-intensity aerobic exercise or 75 minutes of vigorous-intensity aerobic exercise per week, spread across several days.

Intensity: Moderate-intensity activities make you breathe harder and sweat slightly, while vigorous-intensity activities significantly increase heart rate and breathing.

Duration: Sessions should last at least 10 minutes to receive health benefits.

Strength Training: Include strength exercises for all major muscle groups at least twice a week, using weights, resistance bands, or body weight.

Flexibility and Balance: Incorporate stretching and balance exercises into your routine to maintain mobility and prevent injuries.

Getting Started with Exercise:

Consultation: Before starting a new exercise program, consult with a healthcare provider, especially if you have any pre-existing health conditions or concerns.

Progression: Start gradually and increase intensity, duration, and frequency as fitness improves.

Variety: Include different types of exercise to target various aspects of fitness and prevent monotony.

Enjoyment: Choose activities you enjoy and vary your routine to maintain motivation and adherence.

In summary, exercise is essential for promoting physical fitness, maintaining health, and enhancing overall well-being. By incorporating a variety of exercises into a regular routine and following established guidelines, individuals can achieve optimal physical, mental, and emotional health benefits.

Bonus Chapter: Calorie counting

Definition: Calorie counting involves tracking the number of calories consumed from food and beverages throughout the day. The calorie is a unit of energy derived from food and is used by the body for various functions, including metabolism, physical activity, and basic physiological processes.

Purpose:

Weight Management: Calorie counting is commonly used to achieve weight loss, weight maintenance, or weight gain goals by ensuring that calorie intake aligns with caloric expenditure.
Nutrient Awareness: It helps individuals become more aware of their dietary choices and encourages the selection of nutrient-dense foods.
Behavioral Awareness: Tracking calories can promote mindful eating habits, such as recognizing portion sizes and reducing mindless snacking.
Fitness Goals: Athletes and fitness enthusiasts may use calorie counting to support performance goals, such as muscle gain or endurance training.
Basics of Calorie Counting:

Daily Caloric Needs: Calculating daily calorie needs involves considering factors such as age, sex, weight, height, activity level, and goals (e.g., weight loss, maintenance, or gain).
Calorie Intake Tracking: Using food labels, nutrition databases, or mobile apps, individuals track the calories consumed from each food and beverage consumed throughout the day.
Portion Control: Understanding serving sizes and portions is crucial for accurate calorie counting. Measuring food using kitchen scales or measuring cups helps ensure accuracy.
Monitoring Progress: Regularly tracking and reviewing calorie intake helps individuals assess adherence to their calorie goals and adjust as needed.
Components of Calories:

Macronutrients: Calories come from three main macronutrients:
Carbohydrates: Provide 4 calories per gram.
Proteins: Provide 4 calories per gram.
Fats: Provide 9 calories per gram.
Alcohol: Provides 7 calories per gram but is not considered essential for health and should be consumed in moderation.

Challenges and Considerations:

Accuracy: Calorie counting accuracy can vary based on food preparation methods, portion sizes, and individual metabolism.
Nutrient Quality: Focusing solely on calories may overlook the importance of nutrient quality and overall dietary balance.
Behavioral Impact: For some individuals, strict calorie counting can lead to obsessive behaviors or an unhealthy relationship with food.
Individual Variation: Caloric needs and responses to calorie counting can vary widely among individuals based on factors like metabolism, genetics, and health status.
Effective Use:

Setting Realistic Goals: Establishing achievable calorie goals aligned with health and fitness objectives.
Educational Tools: Utilizing nutrition labels, online resources, or mobile apps for accurate calorie information.
Professional Guidance: Seeking advice from registered dietitians or nutritionists for personalized calorie recommendations and support.
In summary, calorie counting is a valuable tool for managing weight, promoting awareness of dietary choices, and supporting various health and fitness goals. When used effectively and with consideration for individual needs and behaviors, calorie counting can contribute to a balanced approach to nutrition and overall well-being.

Bonus Chapter: Body cleansing

Definition: Body cleansing or detoxification refers to the process of eliminating potentially harmful substances, toxins, and waste products from the body. It is believed to enhance the body's natural detoxification mechanisms and support optimal health.

Purpose:

Toxin Removal: The primary goal is to rid the body of accumulated toxins from environmental pollutants, processed foods, medications, and metabolic by-products.

Improved Health: Advocates believe detox programs can improve digestion, boost energy levels, enhance immune function, and promote clearer skin.
Weight Loss: Some detox programs are marketed for weight loss by reducing bloating, water retention, and promoting fat loss.
Resetting Habits: Detox diets often encourage healthier eating habits, increased water intake, and reduced consumption of processed foods, caffeine, and alcohol.
Common Methods of Body Cleansing:

Juice Cleanses: Consuming only fresh fruit and vegetable juices for several days to provide nutrients while reducing the digestive workload.
Fasting: Temporarily abstaining from solid foods or certain types of foods to allow the body to rest and cleanse.
Herbal Supplements: Using herbal teas or supplements purported to support liver function, kidney function, or enhance detoxification processes.
Colon Cleanses: Using enemas, laxatives, or colon hydrotherapy to flush out waste and toxins from the colon.
Saunas and Sweat Therapy: Increasing perspiration through saunas, steam baths, or exercise to eliminate toxins through the skin.
Hydration: Drinking plenty of water and herbal teas to support kidney function and flush out toxins through urination.
Potential Benefits:

Improved Digestion: Eliminating processed foods and stimulating digestion with fiber-rich fruits and vegetables can improve gastrointestinal health.
Increased Energy: Removing toxins that burden the body's systems may lead to increased energy levels and vitality.
Clearer Skin: Detox diets often promote clearer skin by reducing inflammation and improving nutrient absorption.

Mental Clarity: Supporters suggest that detox programs can enhance mental clarity and concentration.
Considerations and Risks:

Nutrient Deficiencies: Some detox programs may lack essential nutrients such as protein, fats, and vitamins, potentially leading to deficiencies if followed long-term.
Potential Side Effects: Detox diets can cause side effects such as fatigue, headaches, dizziness, nausea, or irritability, especially during fasting or drastic dietary changes.
Lack of Scientific Evidence: Scientific research supporting the efficacy and safety of detox diets is limited, and claims about detoxifying specific organs or systems may be unsubstantiated.
Individual Variability: Responses to detox programs vary among individuals, and some may experience negative reactions or worsened health conditions.
Healthy Approaches:

Balanced Diet: Focus on a balanced diet rich in whole foods, fruits, vegetables, lean proteins, and healthy fats to support the body's natural detoxification processes.
Hydration: Drink adequate water daily to support kidney function and flush out toxins through urine.
Regular Exercise: Engage in regular physical activity to promote circulation, lymphatic drainage, and sweat production.
Stress Management: Reduce stress through relaxation techniques, adequate sleep, and mindfulness practices to support overall well-being.

In conclusion, while body cleansing methods are popular for promoting health and vitality, it's essential to approach them with caution and prioritize evidence-based practices that support long-term health and sustainability. Consulting with healthcare professionals, such as registered dietitians or physicians, can provide personalized guidance and ensure safe practices when considering a detox program.

Bonus Chapter: Detoxification

Definition: Detoxification, often abbreviated as detox, refers to the physiological or medicinal removal of toxic substances from the body. It involves the elimination of harmful substances through organs such as the liver, kidneys, lungs, skin, and gastrointestinal tract.

Mechanisms of Detoxification:

Liver Detoxification: The liver plays a central role in detoxification by breaking down toxins into less harmful substances. This process involves two phases: Phase I (oxidation) and Phase II (conjugation), where enzymes transform toxins into water-soluble compounds for excretion.
Kidney Filtration: The kidneys filter blood and excrete waste products and toxins in the form of urine, regulating electrolyte balance and maintaining fluid homeostasis.
Lung Exhalation: The lungs eliminate volatile toxins and metabolic waste products through exhalation, exchanging oxygen and carbon dioxide during respiration.
Skin Secretion: Sweat glands in the skin help eliminate toxins and regulate body temperature. Saunas and sweating therapies promote detoxification through the skin.
Gastrointestinal Elimination: The intestines remove waste and toxins through bowel movements. Fiber-rich foods support regular elimination and bind toxins for excretion.
Natural Detoxification Processes:

Metabolism: Cells continuously undergo metabolic processes that produce waste products, including carbon dioxide, which is expelled through respiration.
Oxidative Stress Response: Antioxidants neutralize free radicals generated during metabolism, reducing oxidative stress and cellular damage.
Immune System Function: Immune cells identify and eliminate pathogens, toxins, and abnormal cells, supporting overall immune function and detoxification.
Lymphatic Drainage: The lymphatic system circulates lymph fluid throughout the body, removing cellular waste and toxins, supporting immune responses and fluid balance.
Detoxification Support:

Nutrition: Consuming a balanced diet rich in antioxidants, vitamins, minerals, and fiber supports liver function and overall detoxification processes. Cruciferous vegetables (e.g., broccoli, kale) and foods high in sulfur compounds (e.g., garlic, onions) promote Phase II detoxification.
Hydration: Drinking an adequate amount of water supports kidney function and facilitates toxin elimination through urine.
Physical Activity: Regular exercise improves circulation, lymphatic drainage, and sweat production, enhancing overall detoxification.
Stress Management: Chronic stress can impair detoxification pathways. Stress reduction techniques such as meditation, yoga, and adequate sleep support overall health and detoxification.
Detoxification Myths:

Detox Diets: Commercial detox diets or cleanses promising rapid toxin elimination may lack scientific evidence and can be restrictive or nutritionally imbalanced.
Supplements: Detox supplements or herbal remedies claiming to cleanse specific organs (e.g., liver detox supplements) may not have sufficient scientific backing and should be used with caution.
Prolonged Fasting: Extended fasting or extreme dietary restrictions for detoxification purposes can lead to nutrient deficiencies and metabolic imbalances.
Clinical Detoxification:

Medical Detox: In clinical settings, detoxification refers to the supervised withdrawal from drugs or alcohol to manage withdrawal symptoms and prevent complications.
Environmental Toxins: Occupational or environmental exposure to toxins may require medical intervention, such as chelation therapy to remove heavy metals.

In conclusion, detoxification is a vital physiological process that supports overall health by eliminating toxins and metabolic waste products. Supporting natural detoxification pathways through a balanced diet, hydration, regular exercise, and stress management promotes optimal health and well-being. It's essential to approach detoxification with evidence-based practices and consult healthcare professionals for personalized guidance, especially when considering detox programs or therapies.

Bonus Chapter: Hiit

Definition: HIIT is a form of cardiovascular exercise strategy alternating short bursts of intense anaerobic exercise (high-intensity intervals) with less intense recovery periods (low-intensity intervals or rest). This cyclical pattern challenges both aerobic and anaerobic energy systems, promoting significant physiological adaptations.

Key Components:

Intensity: High-intensity intervals typically range from 80% to 95% of an individual's maximum heart rate or perceived exertion, often described as "pushing to the limit."
Duration: Intervals typically last from 20 seconds to 2 minutes, followed by recovery periods lasting 1 to 2 times the length of the high-intensity segment.
Recovery: Low-intensity intervals or complete rest periods allow for partial or complete recovery of energy stores and physiological systems before the next intense effort.
Benefits of HIIT:

Efficiency: HIIT sessions are usually shorter (10-30 minutes) compared to traditional aerobic workouts while delivering comparable or superior cardiovascular and metabolic benefits.
Fat Burning: HIIT increases metabolism and promotes fat oxidation during and after exercise, contributing to weight loss and fat loss.
Cardiovascular Fitness: Improves aerobic capacity (VO2 max), cardiac function, and endurance due to the demanding nature of intense intervals.
Muscle Strength: HIIT incorporates bodyweight exercises or resistance training, enhancing muscle strength and power.
Metabolic Health: Enhances insulin sensitivity, glucose regulation, and lipid profiles, potentially reducing the risk of metabolic disorders like type 2 diabetes.
EPOC (Excess Post-Exercise Oxygen Consumption): HIIT stimulates EPOC, causing the body to consume additional oxygen post-exercise to restore physiological functions, leading to increased calorie expenditure.
Time Efficiency: Suitable for individuals with busy schedules who seek effective workouts within limited time frames.
Types of HIIT Workouts:

Tabata: A specific HIIT protocol involving 20 seconds of ultra-intense exercise followed by 10 seconds of rest, repeated for 4 minutes (8 rounds).

Interval Training: Varied intervals combining sprinting, cycling, rowing, or bodyweight exercises with active recovery periods.

Circuit Training: Incorporates multiple exercises targeting different muscle groups, rotating between stations with minimal rest.

Considerations:

Safety: HIIT should be tailored to individual fitness levels and health conditions. Beginners or those with medical concerns should start with low-intensity intervals and gradually increase intensity and duration.

Recovery: Adequate rest and recovery between HIIT sessions are crucial to prevent overtraining and promote muscle repair and growth.

Progression: Gradually increase intensity, duration, or complexity of intervals as fitness improves to continually challenge the body and avoid plateauing.

Implementation:

Warm-Up: Always begin with a dynamic warm-up to prepare muscles, joints, and cardiovascular system for intense exercise.

Cool Down: Conclude with a cooldown period involving stretching and deep breathing to promote muscle relaxation and reduce post-exercise soreness.

Frequency: Incorporate HIIT workouts into a balanced exercise routine, combining with strength training, flexibility exercises, and low-impact aerobic activities for comprehensive fitness benefits.

In summary, HIIT is a highly effective exercise strategy offering diverse benefits in a time-efficient manner. When performed safely and progressively, HIIT can significantly enhance cardiovascular fitness, metabolic health, and overall well-being, making it suitable for various fitness levels and goals.

Bonus Chapter: Detoxification lifestyle

Definition: A detoxification lifestyle encompasses daily practices, dietary choices, and behavioral habits aimed at minimizing toxin exposure, supporting organ function, and enhancing the body's ability to eliminate toxins effectively.

Key Components:

Nutrient-Dense Diet: Emphasizes whole, unprocessed foods rich in vitamins, minerals, antioxidants, and fiber to support liver and kidney function. Examples include fruits, vegetables, whole grains, lean proteins, and healthy fats.

Hydration: Drinking an adequate amount of water daily (approximately 8 glasses or 2 liters) supports kidney function and facilitates the elimination of toxins through urine.

Physical Activity: Regular exercise, including cardiovascular workouts, strength training, and flexibility exercises, enhances circulation, lymphatic drainage, and sweat production, promoting detoxification through the skin and respiratory system.

Stress Management: Chronic stress can impair detoxification pathways. Techniques such as meditation, yoga, deep breathing exercises, and adequate sleep support relaxation, hormone balance, and overall well-being.

Avoidance of Toxins: Minimizing exposure to environmental toxins, pollutants, and synthetic chemicals found in processed foods, pesticides, personal care products, and household cleaners reduces the body's toxin burden.

Sauna Therapy: Utilizing infrared saunas or steam rooms to induce sweating and facilitate the elimination of toxins through the skin.

Quality Sleep: Adequate sleep (7-9 hours per night) supports cellular repair, hormone balance, and cognitive function, essential for overall health and detoxification.

Detoxification Supportive Practices:

Intermittent Fasting: Incorporating periods of fasting or reduced calorie intake may enhance cellular repair processes and promote autophagy, a cellular cleansing mechanism.

Herbal Supplements: Certain herbs and botanicals, such as milk thistle, dandelion root, and turmeric, are believed to support liver function and aid in detoxification. However, their efficacy and safety should be assessed with professional guidance.

Colon Cleansing: Practitioners may utilize enemas, colon hydrotherapy, or dietary fiber supplements to promote regular bowel movements and eliminate waste products from the colon.

Mindful Eating: Practicing mindful eating habits, such as chewing food thoroughly, eating slowly, and paying attention to hunger cues, supports digestion, nutrient absorption, and overall gastrointestinal health.

Benefits of a Detoxification Lifestyle:

Improved Energy Levels: By reducing toxin exposure and supporting organ function, individuals often report increased energy, vitality, and mental clarity.

Enhanced Immune Function: A well-supported detoxification lifestyle can strengthen the immune system's ability to defend against infections and disease.

Weight Management: Supporting metabolic processes and reducing inflammation through healthy lifestyle practices can contribute to weight loss or maintenance goals.

Clearer Skin: Reduced toxin exposure and improved nutrient intake can promote clearer, healthier skin.

Considerations:

Individual Variability: The effectiveness and safety of detoxification practices may vary among individuals based on age, health status, medications, and genetic factors.

Professional Guidance: Consulting with healthcare professionals, such as registered dietitians, naturopathic doctors, or integrative medicine practitioners, can provide personalized recommendations and ensure safe implementation of detoxification strategies.

Balanced Approach: Adopting a balanced detoxification lifestyle involves integrating evidence-based practices with individual preferences and needs, avoiding extreme or unsustainable measures.

In conclusion, a detoxification lifestyle encompasses holistic practices that support the body's natural detoxification mechanisms, promoting optimal health and vitality. By focusing on nutrient-dense foods, hydration, physical activity, stress management, and toxin avoidance, individuals can enhance their overall well-being and reduce the burden of toxins on the body.

Bonus Chapter: Detox benefits

Enhanced Liver Function: The liver is a crucial organ involved in detoxification processes, breaking down toxins and metabolic waste products. Supporting liver function through a balanced diet rich in antioxidants, vitamins, and minerals can enhance its ability to metabolize and eliminate toxins effectively.

Reduced Inflammation: Chronic inflammation is linked to numerous health conditions, including cardiovascular disease, diabetes, and autoimmune disorders. Detox diets emphasizing anti-inflammatory foods such as fruits, vegetables, and omega-3 fatty acids may help reduce systemic inflammation levels.

Improved Digestive Health: Detox diets often focus on fiber-rich foods and adequate hydration, promoting regular bowel movements and supporting gastrointestinal health. Fiber helps eliminate waste and toxins from the colon, reducing the risk of constipation and promoting gut flora balance.

Increased Energy Levels: Advocates of detox diets often report feeling more energetic and alert following a cleanse. This can be attributed to reduced toxin load, improved nutrient absorption, and enhanced metabolic efficiency.

Weight Loss: Short-term detox programs may lead to weight loss due to reduced calorie intake, increased water loss, and improved metabolism. However, long-term weight management requires sustainable dietary and lifestyle changes beyond detox periods.

Clearer Skin: Detox diets advocating for the elimination of processed foods, sugars, and artificial additives may result in clearer skin. Improved hydration, balanced hormone levels, and reduced inflammation contribute to healthier skin appearance.

Enhanced Mental Clarity: Some individuals report improved mental focus and clarity during and after detox diets. This may be attributed to reduced toxin exposure, balanced blood sugar levels, and the promotion of brain-healthy nutrients.

Support for Healthy Aging: Detox diets rich in antioxidants and anti-inflammatory compounds may support cellular repair processes and protect against oxidative stress, potentially slowing down the aging process and promoting longevity.

Immune System Support: A well-balanced diet supporting detoxification processes can strengthen the immune system by reducing the body's toxic burden and promoting optimal organ function.

Behavioral Changes: Participating in a detox program often encourages individuals to adopt healthier eating habits, increase physical activity, and reduce exposure to environmental toxins, fostering long-term lifestyle changes.

While these potential benefits are frequently reported anecdotally, it's important to note that scientific evidence supporting the efficacy and long-term benefits of detox diets varies. The body's natural detoxification mechanisms are robust, and maintaining a balanced diet rich in whole foods, staying hydrated, regular exercise, and stress management are essential for supporting overall health and well-being. Consulting with healthcare professionals before embarking on any detox program is advisable, especially for individuals with underlying health conditions or specific dietary needs.

Bonus Chapter: Detoxification recipes

Emphasis on Whole Foods: Detox recipes prioritize fresh, unprocessed ingredients such as fruits, vegetables, whole grains, lean proteins, nuts, seeds, and healthy fats. These foods are rich in vitamins, minerals, antioxidants, and fiber, essential for supporting detoxification pathways in the body.

Antioxidant-Rich Ingredients: Antioxidants play a crucial role in neutralizing free radicals and reducing oxidative stress, which can damage cells and tissues. Recipes often include colorful fruits and vegetables like berries, leafy greens, citrus fruits, and cruciferous vegetables (e.g., broccoli, kale) known for their high antioxidant content.

Hydration: Adequate hydration supports detoxification by promoting kidney function and aiding in the elimination of toxins through urine. Detox recipes may include herbal teas, infused water with lemon or cucumber, and hydrating soups to enhance fluid intake.

Detoxifying Herbs and Spices: Certain herbs and spices are believed to support liver detoxification processes. Common additions include turmeric (with its active compound curcumin), ginger, garlic, cilantro, parsley, and dandelion root, known for their potential detoxifying and anti-inflammatory properties.

Fiber-Rich Foods: Fiber supports digestive health and regular bowel movements, aiding in the elimination of waste and toxins from the body. Detox recipes often incorporate whole grains (e.g., quinoa, brown rice), legumes (e.g., lentils, beans), and fibrous fruits and vegetables to promote gastrointestinal function.

Lean Proteins: High-quality proteins such as lean poultry, fish, tofu, and legumes provide essential amino acids for cellular repair and support muscle function during detoxification.

Avoidance of Processed Foods and Sugars: Detox recipes exclude processed foods, refined sugars, artificial additives, and trans fats, which can contribute to inflammation and hinder detoxification processes.

Balanced Macronutrients: Recipes aim to maintain a balanced ratio of macronutrients (carbohydrates, proteins, and fats) to support energy levels, stabilize blood sugar, and promote satiety.

Cooking Methods: Recipes often favor steaming, sautéing with healthy oils (e.g., olive oil, coconut oil), baking, or raw preparations to preserve nutrient content and minimize added fats and sodium.

Sample Detox Recipes:

Detox Smoothie: Blend spinach, kale, berries, avocado, and almond milk with a scoop of plant-based protein powder.
Quinoa Salad: Combine cooked quinoa with cucumber, tomatoes, bell peppers, parsley, lemon juice, and a drizzle of olive oil.
Herbal Detox Tea: Steep ginger, turmeric, lemon slices, and mint leaves in hot water for a refreshing beverage.
When preparing detox recipes, it's essential to focus on variety, moderation, and individual dietary preferences or restrictions. While these recipes are nutrient-dense and supportive of overall health, consulting with a healthcare professional or registered dietitian is recommended, especially for individuals with specific health concerns or medical conditions. This ensures that detox programs are safe, effective, and tailored to individual needs for long-term health benefits.

Bonus Chapter: Detoxification plan

A detoxification plan, often referred to as a detox plan or cleanse, is a structured approach aimed at supporting the body's natural detoxification processes to eliminate toxins, promote overall health, and potentially achieve specific health goals. Here's a detailed explanation of what a detoxification plan typically involves:

Goal Setting: A detox plan begins with setting clear goals, whether it's to boost energy levels, support weight loss, improve digestive health, enhance skin clarity, or reduce inflammation. Clear objectives help tailor the plan to individual needs and track progress effectively.

Duration: Detox plans can vary in duration, ranging from a few days to several weeks, depending on the specific goals, individual health status, and type of detox program chosen.

Types of Detox Plans:

Whole Foods-Based Detox: Focuses on eliminating processed foods, sugars, alcohol, caffeine, and additives, while emphasizing nutrient-dense whole foods such as fruits, vegetables, lean proteins, whole grains, nuts, and seeds.

Juice Cleanses: Involves consuming freshly squeezed juices from fruits and vegetables for a period, providing concentrated vitamins, minerals, and antioxidants while reducing fiber intake.

Elimination Diets: Temporarily excludes potential allergens or sensitivities like gluten, dairy, soy, or specific food groups to identify triggers and support gut health.

Water Fasting: Restricts caloric intake to water only for a short period, promoting autophagy (cellular repair) and metabolic cleansing.

Supplemented Detox: Incorporates specific herbs, supplements, or detoxifying drinks to support liver function, enhance bile production, or promote bowel movements.

Intermittent Fasting: Alternates between periods of eating and fasting, promoting cellular repair processes and metabolic flexibility.

Medical Supervised Detox: Administered under healthcare provider supervision, often for severe toxin exposure or substance abuse recovery.

Components of a Detoxification Plan:

Nutrient-Dense Foods: Emphasizes whole, unprocessed foods rich in antioxidants, vitamins, minerals, and fiber to support organ function and promote toxin elimination.

Hydration: Encourages adequate water intake to support kidney function and enhance toxin elimination through urine.

Physical Activity: Includes regular exercise to support circulation, lymphatic drainage, and sweat production, facilitating toxin release through the skin.

Stress Management: Incorporates stress-reducing practices such as meditation, deep breathing exercises, or yoga to support hormone balance and overall well-being.

Sleep Optimization: Promotes sufficient sleep duration and quality to facilitate cellular repair, hormone regulation, and cognitive function.

Toxin Avoidance: Minimizes exposure to environmental toxins, pollutants, and synthetic chemicals found in food, water, personal care products, and household cleaners.

Monitoring and Adjustments: Throughout the detox plan, monitoring progress, symptoms, and overall well-being is essential. Adjustments may be made based on individual responses, ensuring the detox program remains safe, effective, and sustainable.

Post-Detox Transition: Gradual reintroduction of eliminated foods or gradual return to regular eating patterns is crucial to maintain the benefits achieved during the detox period. Adopting healthy eating habits and lifestyle practices long-term supports continued health benefits.

Considerations:

Individualization: Detox plans should be tailored to individual health needs, preferences, and medical conditions. Consulting with a healthcare professional or registered dietitian is recommended, especially before starting a more restrictive detox program.

Safety: Some detox methods, such as extended fasting or intense cleansing regimens, may not be suitable for everyone, particularly those with underlying health conditions, pregnant or breastfeeding women, or individuals with eating disorders.

Long-Term Benefits: While short-term detox plans may provide immediate benefits such as increased energy and improved digestion, maintaining a balanced diet, regular physical activity, and healthy lifestyle habits are key for long-term health and well-being.

In conclusion, a well-designed detoxification plan can support the body's natural detox processes, enhance overall health, and help achieve specific health goals when implemented safely and effectively. Understanding the principles and components of detox plans allows individuals to make informed decisions and optimize their health journey.

Bonus Chapter: Detoxification process

Liver Detoxification: The liver is the primary organ responsible for detoxifying chemicals, drugs, and metabolic byproducts from the bloodstream. It processes toxins into less harmful substances through two main phases:

Phase I: Enzymes in the liver convert fat-soluble toxins into intermediate metabolites.
Phase II: These metabolites are further processed and conjugated with water-soluble substances, making them easier to excrete via bile or urine.
Kidney Filtration: The kidneys filter blood and remove water-soluble waste products, toxins, and excess substances like electrolytes and urea from the body through urine. Adequate hydration supports kidney function in flushing out toxins effectively.

Gastrointestinal Tract: The digestive system plays a crucial role in detoxification by processing nutrients and eliminating waste products. The colon absorbs water and minerals from digested food while eliminating undigested materials and toxins through bowel movements.

Lymphatic System: The lymphatic system circulates lymph fluid throughout the body, collecting and removing cellular waste, toxins, and pathogens. Physical activity supports lymphatic drainage, aiding in toxin elimination.

Skin Detoxification: Sweat glands in the skin help eliminate water-soluble toxins, salts, and heavy metals through perspiration. Saunas and regular exercise promote sweating, aiding in skin detoxification.

Respiratory System: The lungs eliminate gaseous waste products like carbon dioxide through respiration. Deep breathing exercises and maintaining good air quality support lung function in eliminating toxins.

Antioxidant Defense: Antioxidants such as vitamins C and E, glutathione, and enzymes like superoxide dismutase (SOD) neutralize free radicals generated during detoxification processes, reducing oxidative stress and cellular damage.

Role of Nutrients: Essential nutrients like B vitamins, magnesium, zinc, and amino acids are cofactors in detoxification enzyme pathways. Consuming a balanced diet rich in these nutrients supports efficient detoxification processes.

Detoxification Phases: The detoxification process occurs in phases, starting with recognition and mobilization of toxins, followed by transformation and conjugation in the liver, and finally excretion via urine, bile, sweat, or feces.

Factors Affecting Detoxification: Individual factors such as genetics, age, diet, lifestyle habits, environmental exposures, and underlying health conditions influence detoxification efficiency. Optimizing these factors through healthy lifestyle choices supports overall detoxification.

Detoxification Support: Techniques like intermittent fasting, herbal supplementation, periodic cleansing diets, and lifestyle practices such as stress management, adequate hydration, and regular exercise can enhance detoxification pathways and support overall health.

Understanding the complex interplay of organs, systems, nutrients, and lifestyle factors involved in detoxification helps individuals make informed decisions about supporting their body's natural detox processes for improved health and well-being. Consulting with healthcare professionals or registered dietitians can provide personalized guidance on safe and effective detox strategies tailored to individual needs.

Bonus Chapter: Bodyweight exercises

Bodyweight exercises are physical activities that use the body's own weight as resistance to build strength, endurance, flexibility, and coordination. These exercises are versatile and effective, requiring minimal to no equipment, making them accessible for people of various fitness levels and settings. Here's an expert explanation of bodyweight exercises, their benefits, and examples:

Benefits of Bodyweight Exercises:
Convenience and Accessibility: Bodyweight exercises can be performed anywhere, such as at home, in a park, or while traveling, without the need for gym equipment. This accessibility makes it easier to maintain a consistent fitness routine.

Cost-Effective: They require minimal or no equipment, reducing costs associated with gym memberships or purchasing fitness gear.

Functional Strength: Bodyweight exercises engage multiple muscle groups simultaneously, improving overall strength and coordination that translates to better performance in daily activities and sports.

Versatility: There are countless variations and progressions of bodyweight exercises, allowing for customization based on fitness goals, skill levels, and specific muscle groups targeted.

Balance and Stability: Many bodyweight exercises engage core muscles and stabilizers to maintain balance and control, enhancing overall stability and reducing the risk of injuries.

Scalability: Bodyweight exercises can be adapted for beginners to advanced fitness levels by adjusting repetitions, intensity, range of motion, and incorporating variations like plyometrics or isometric holds.

Examples of Bodyweight Exercises:
Upper Body Exercises:

Push-Ups: Strengthen chest, shoulders, and triceps.
Pull-Ups/Chin-Ups: Target back, biceps, and core.
Dips: Focus on triceps, shoulders, and chest.
Lower Body Exercises:

Squats: Work quadriceps, hamstrings, glutes, and calves.
Lunges: Engage quads, hamstrings, and glutes.
Step-Ups: Strengthen legs and improve balance.
Core Exercises:

Plank Variations: Engage entire core, including abdominals, obliques, and lower back.
Mountain Climbers: Work core and cardio endurance.
Leg Raises: Target lower abdominals and hip flexors.
Total Body Exercises:

Burpees: Combine cardio, strength, and full-body coordination.

Bear Crawls: Enhance coordination, core strength, and endurance.

Bodyweight Rows: Engage back, biceps, and core.

Programming Bodyweight Exercises:

Warm-Up: Perform dynamic stretches or light cardio to prepare muscles and joints.

Workout Structure: Design a circuit or use interval training (e.g., Tabata) with bodyweight exercises to optimize cardiovascular fitness and muscular endurance.

Progression: Gradually increase repetitions, intensity (e.g., adding plyometric jumps), or complexity (e.g., one-arm push-ups) to challenge muscles and prevent plateau.

Safety Considerations:

Proper Form: Maintain proper alignment and technique to reduce injury risk and maximize effectiveness.

Rest and Recovery: Allow adequate rest between sessions to prevent overtraining and promote muscle repair.

Consultation: Individuals with pre-existing conditions or beginners should consult with a fitness professional or healthcare provider before starting a new exercise program.

Bodyweight exercises offer a flexible and effective way to improve fitness, build strength, and enhance overall health without requiring specialized equipment. Integrating these exercises into a balanced fitness routine alongside proper nutrition and hydration supports long-term wellness and physical performance.

More Bonus I

Weightlifting
Definition: Weightlifting involves lifting weights, such as barbells, dumbbells, or kettlebells, to build strength, muscle mass, and power.

Benefits:

Strength Gain: Increases muscle strength and size through progressive overload.
Bone Health: Stimulates bone density and reduces the risk of osteoporosis.
Metabolism: Boosts metabolism, aiding in weight management.
Functional Strength: Enhances daily activities and sports performance.
Considerations:

Form and Technique: Proper form is crucial to prevent injuries.
Progression: Gradually increase weight and intensity for continuous gains.
Rest and Recovery: Muscles need time to repair and grow between sessions.
Cardio

Definition: Cardiovascular exercise, or cardio, involves activities that increase heart rate and oxygen consumption, improving cardiovascular health and endurance.

Benefits:

Heart Health: Strengthens the heart muscle and improves circulation.
Calorie Burn: Helps burn calories and support weight loss.
Endurance: Enhances stamina and oxygen efficiency.
Mood Enhancement: Releases endorphins, reducing stress and improving mood.
Types:

Running, Cycling, Swimming: Continuous aerobic activities.
HIIT (High-Intensity Interval Training): Alternates between intense bursts and recovery periods.
Aerobic Classes: Dance-based or step workouts.
Strength Training
Definition: Strength training involves resistance exercises to build muscle strength, power, and endurance using bodyweight, free weights, or resistance machines.

Benefits:

Muscle Development: Increases muscle mass and definition.
Metabolism: Boosts metabolism for fat loss and weight management.
Joint Health: Strengthens connective tissues and supports joint function.
Balance and Stability: Improves posture, coordination, and functional movements.
Methods:

Free Weights: Dumbbells, barbells, kettlebells.
Machines: Guided resistance exercises.

Bodyweight: Push-ups, squats, planks.
Yoga
Definition: Yoga is a mind-body practice that combines physical postures, breathing techniques, and meditation or relaxation to enhance physical and mental well-being.

Benefits:

Flexibility: Improves range of motion and joint mobility.
Strength: Builds core strength and muscular endurance.
Stress Reduction: Promotes relaxation and reduces anxiety.
Mindfulness: Enhances focus, concentration, and self-awareness.
Types:

Hatha: Gentle practice with basic poses.
Vinyasa: Flowing sequences synchronized with breath.
Bikram/Hot Yoga: Practiced in a heated room.
Yin: Passive poses held for longer durations.
Pilates
Definition: Pilates is a low-impact exercise method that focuses on core strength, flexibility, and alignment through controlled movements.

Benefits:

Core Strength: Targets deep abdominal muscles (transverse abdominis).
Posture: Improves alignment and spinal mobility.
Flexibility: Enhances muscle elasticity and joint range of motion.
Injury Prevention: Develops balanced muscle strength to prevent injuries.
Equipment:

Mat Pilates: Bodyweight exercises on a mat.

Reformer Pilates: Uses a machine with springs for resistance.
Props: Resistance bands, balls, and circles for added challenge.
CrossFit
Definition: CrossFit is a high-intensity fitness program that incorporates functional movements, Olympic weightlifting, and cardiovascular exercises performed in varied workouts.

Benefits:

Overall Fitness: Improves strength, endurance, flexibility, and agility.
Community: Fosters camaraderie and motivation through group classes.
Adaptability: Scales workouts for different fitness levels and abilities.
Components:

Workouts of the Day (WOD): Daily varied routines.
Functional Movements: Squats, deadlifts, pulls, and presses.
Intensity: Emphasizes speed, power, and endurance in short, intense workouts.
Kettlebells
Definition: Kettlebells are cast-iron weights with a handle used for ballistic exercises that combine cardiovascular, strength, and flexibility training.

Benefits:

Cardiovascular Fitness: Improves heart health and endurance.
Strength Development: Builds muscle strength and power.
Core Stability: Engages core muscles for balance and control.
Versatility: Allows for dynamic movements and full-body workouts.
Exercises:

Swings: Hip hinge movement for power and conditioning.

Turkish Get-Up: Full-body exercise for strength and stability.
Snatches: Explosive movement for power and coordination.
Resistance Bands
Definition: Resistance bands are elastic bands used for strength training, stretching, and rehabilitation exercises to provide resistance without weights.

Benefits:

Portability: Lightweight and compact for travel and home workouts.
Versatility: Offers variable resistance levels for different muscle groups.
Rehabilitation: Supports gentle strengthening and flexibility exercises.
Muscle Activation: Enhances muscle recruitment and endurance.
Exercises:

Banded Squats: Adds resistance to lower body movements.
Rows: Targets back and shoulder muscles.
Stretching: Assists in deepening stretches and improving flexibility.
Stretching
Definition: Stretching exercises aim to improve flexibility, range of motion, and muscle elasticity through lengthening and elongating muscle fibers.

Benefits:

Flexibility: Increases joint mobility and range of motion.
Injury Prevention: Reduces muscle tension and risk of strains.
Recovery: Promotes circulation and muscle relaxation post-exercise.
Posture: Improves alignment and reduces muscle imbalances.
Types:

Static Stretching: Hold positions to stretch muscles passively.
Dynamic Stretching: Incorporates movement to warm up muscles.
Proprioceptive Neuromuscular Facilitation (PNF): Combines passive stretching and isometric contractions for enhanced flexibility.
Home Workouts
Definition: Home workouts are exercise routines performed at home using minimal equipment or bodyweight exercises.

Benefits:

Convenience: Eliminates travel time to gyms or fitness studios.
Cost-Effective: Saves money on gym memberships and commuting.
Privacy: Allows for personalized workouts in a comfortable environment.
Flexibility: Offers scheduling flexibility to fit workouts into daily routines.
Equipment:

Bodyweight: Push-ups, squats, lunges, planks.
Minimal Equipment: Resistance bands, dumbbells, yoga mat.
Online Resources: Access to virtual classes, workout apps, and streaming platforms.
Gym Routines
Definition: Gym routines are structured exercise programs performed at fitness centers using a variety of equipment and facilities.

Benefits:

Equipment Variety: Access to cardio machines, free weights, resistance machines, and specialized equipment.

Expert Guidance: Support from fitness professionals, trainers, and group instructors.
Motivation: Surroundings and peers can encourage adherence to fitness goals.
Progress Tracking: Facilities often offer fitness assessments and tracking tools.
Components:

Warm-Up: Cardiovascular activity or dynamic stretches.
Strength Training: Using free weights, machines, or bodyweight exercises.
Cardiovascular Exercise: Treadmills, ellipticals, bikes, or group classes.
Cool-Down: Gentle stretching or foam rolling to aid in recovery.
Each of these fitness categories offers unique benefits and considerations, catering to different preferences, fitness levels, and goals. Integrating a variety of exercises and modalities into a balanced fitness routine promotes overall health, strength, endurance, and well-being. For personalized guidance or program development, consulting with fitness professionals or certified trainers can provide tailored recommendations aligned with individual needs and objectives.

More Bonus II

Portion Control
Definition: Portion control involves managing the amount of food consumed in a single sitting or throughout the day to regulate calorie intake.

Importance:

Calorie Management: Prevents overeating and supports weight management goals.
Nutrient Balance: Ensures a balanced intake of macronutrients (carbohydrates, proteins, fats) and micronutrients (vitamins, minerals).
Healthy Habits: Promotes mindful eating and awareness of portion sizes.
Practical Tips:

Use smaller plates and bowls to control portions visually.
Measure serving sizes using cups, spoons, or scales.
Practice mindful eating by savoring each bite and eating slowly.
Balanced Diet
Definition: A balanced diet includes a variety of foods from all food groups in appropriate proportions to meet nutritional needs for optimal health and well-being.

Components:

Fruits and Vegetables: Rich in vitamins, minerals, and fiber.
Proteins: Lean meats, poultry, fish, beans, and legumes.
Whole Grains: Brown rice, quinoa, whole wheat pasta for complex carbohydrates.
Dairy or Alternatives: Low-fat dairy, fortified soy milk for calcium and vitamin D.
Healthy Fats: Olive oil, nuts, seeds for essential fatty acids.
Benefits:

Provides essential nutrients for energy, growth, and repair.
Supports immune function, bone health, and overall vitality.
Reduces the risk of chronic diseases like heart disease and diabetes.
Low Calorie
Definition: A low-calorie diet restricts daily calorie intake to promote weight loss or manage weight by creating a calorie deficit.

Purpose:

Weight Loss: Consuming fewer calories than the body burns promotes fat loss.
Calorie Control: Increases awareness of calorie content in foods.
Health Benefits: May improve metabolic health and reduce disease risk factors.
Caution:

Ensure adequate nutrition despite calorie restriction.
Monitor energy levels and physical activity to prevent nutrient deficiencies.
Consult with a healthcare professional for personalized guidance.
High Protein

Definition: A high-protein diet emphasizes increased intake of protein-rich foods to support muscle growth, repair, and overall health.

Benefits:

Muscle Maintenance: Supports muscle mass and strength, especially during exercise and aging.
Satiety: Helps control appetite and reduce cravings, aiding in weight management.
Metabolic Health: Supports metabolism, hormone production, and immune function.
Sources:

Lean meats, poultry, fish, eggs, dairy products for animal-based proteins.
Beans, legumes, tofu, tempeh, quinoa for plant-based proteins.
Considerations:

Balance protein intake with carbohydrates and fats for a well-rounded diet.
Drink plenty of water to support kidney function when consuming higher protein amounts.
Low Carb
Definition: A low-carb diet restricts carbohydrate intake, typically emphasizing protein and fat consumption, to promote weight loss or manage conditions like diabetes.

Purpose:

Blood Sugar Control: Reduces blood glucose spikes and insulin levels.
Weight Loss: Promotes fat burning and reduces appetite.
Metabolic Health: Improves cholesterol levels and cardiovascular health markers.
Foods to Limit:

Sugar-sweetened beverages, refined grains, processed foods.
Emphasize non-starchy vegetables, lean proteins, healthy fats.
Individualization:

Adjust carbohydrate intake based on activity level, health goals, and metabolic needs.
Monitor nutrient intake to ensure dietary balance and long-term sustainability.
Low Fat
Definition: A low-fat diet reduces fat intake, particularly saturated and trans fats, to support heart health and weight management.

Purpose:

Heart Health: Lowers cholesterol levels and reduces the risk of heart disease.
Weight Management: Reduces calorie intake from fats, which are more calorie-dense than carbohydrates or proteins.
Digestive Health: Supports gallbladder function and digestion.
Sources:

Choose lean meats, poultry without skin, fish, low-fat dairy products.
Include plant-based fats like avocados, nuts, seeds, and olive oil in moderation.
Balanced Approach:

Focus on healthy fats and limit unhealthy fats.
Emphasize whole foods and minimize processed foods with added fats and sugars.
Vegetarian Diet

Definition: A vegetarian diet excludes meat and seafood but may include dairy products and eggs, focusing on plant-based foods for nutrition.

Types:

Lacto-Ovo Vegetarian: Includes dairy and eggs.
Lacto-Vegetarian: Includes dairy but excludes eggs.
Ovo-Vegetarian: Includes eggs but excludes dairy.
Vegan: Excludes all animal products, including dairy, eggs, and honey.
Benefits:

Nutrient-Rich: Rich in vitamins, minerals, fiber, and antioxidants from plant sources.
Heart Health: Lower saturated fat and cholesterol intake may reduce heart disease risk.
Environmental Impact: Promotes sustainability and reduces carbon footprint.
Considerations:

Ensure adequate protein, vitamin B12, iron, zinc, and omega-3 fatty acids through plant-based sources or supplements.
Plan meals to meet nutritional needs and maintain balanced energy levels.
Vegan Diet
Definition: A vegan diet excludes all animal products, including meat, dairy, eggs, and honey, focusing on plant-based foods for nutrition.

Benefits:

Plant-Based Nutrition: High in fiber, vitamins, minerals, and phytonutrients.
Heart Health: Lowers cholesterol levels and reduces the risk of heart disease.

Environmental Sustainability: Supports ethical and sustainable food choices.
Sources:

Legumes, tofu, tempeh, nuts, seeds for protein.
Fortified plant milks, cereals, nutritional yeast for vitamin B12.
Leafy greens, beans, fortified foods for iron and calcium.
Supplementation:

Consider vitamin B12, vitamin D, omega-3 fatty acids, and iron supplements as needed.
Plan meals to ensure adequate protein and nutrient intake for optimal health.
Mediterranean Diet
Definition: The Mediterranean diet is inspired by traditional eating habits of countries bordering the Mediterranean Sea, emphasizing whole foods and healthy fats.

Components:

Plant-Based Foods: Fruits, vegetables, whole grains, legumes, nuts, seeds.
Healthy Fats: Olive oil, nuts, seeds, avocados, fatty fish (e.g., salmon, sardines).
Moderate Dairy: Greek yogurt, cheese.
Lean Proteins: Poultry, eggs, legumes.
Occasional Red Wine: In moderation.
Benefits:

Heart Health: Reduces risk factors for heart disease, such as cholesterol and blood pressure.
Antioxidants: Rich in antioxidants, reducing inflammation and oxidative stress.
Longevity: Associated with lower rates of chronic diseases and improved longevity.
Adherence:

Emphasize whole, minimally processed foods and fresh ingredients.
Incorporate herbs and spices for flavor and added health benefits.
Ketogenic Diet
Definition: The ketogenic (keto) diet is a low-carbohydrate, high-fat diet that induces ketosis, a metabolic state where the body burns fat for fuel instead of carbohydrates.

Purpose:

Weight Loss: Promotes fat burning and reduces appetite.
Blood Sugar Control: Stabilizes blood glucose levels and insulin sensitivity.
Brain Health: May support cognitive function and epilepsy management.
Macronutrient Ratio:

High fat (70-80% of total calories), moderate protein (20-25%), very low carb (5-10%).
Foods to Include:

Healthy fats (avocados, nuts, seeds, olive oil).
Moderate protein (meat, poultry, fish, eggs).
Non-starchy vegetables (leafy greens, broccoli, cauliflower).
Monitoring:

Monitor ketone levels through blood, urine, or breath tests.
Maintain hydration and electrolyte balance, especially during initial adaptation.
Intermittent Fasting
Definition: Intermittent fasting (IF) involves cycling between periods of eating and fasting to promote metabolic health, weight loss, and cellular repair.

Methods:

16/8 Method: Daily fasting for 16 hours, eating within an 8-hour window.
5:2 Diet: Regular eating for 5 days, limited calorie intake (500-600 calories) on 2 non-consecutive days.
Alternate-Day Fasting: Alternating between fasting days and eating days.
Benefits:

Weight Loss: Reduces calorie intake and promotes fat burning.
Insulin Sensitivity: Improves blood sugar control and insulin sensitivity.
Cellular Repair: Enhances autophagy, the process of cellular cleansing and repair.
Adherence:

Stay hydrated and focus on nutrient-dense foods during eating periods.
Monitor hunger cues and adjust fasting schedules to individual preferences and lifestyle.
Clean Eating
Definition: Clean eating emphasizes whole, minimally processed foods while reducing or avoiding processed foods, additives, and artificial ingredients.

Principles:

Whole Foods: Choose natural, unprocessed foods in their original state.
Nutrient Density: Opt for foods rich in vitamins, minerals, and antioxidants.
Hydration: Drink plenty of water and limit sugary beverages.
Mindful Eating: Pay attention to hunger cues and eating habits.

Foods to Enjoy:

Fresh fruits and vegetables.
Whole grains (quinoa, brown rice).
Lean proteins (chicken, fish, legumes).
Healthy fats (avocado)

More Bonus III

Bodybuilding
Definition: Bodybuilding is a discipline focused on developing
and sculpting muscles through resistance training, nutrition,
and supplementation.

Key Aspects:

Resistance Training: Emphasizes lifting weights to increase
muscle size and strength.
Nutrition: High-protein diet to support muscle repair and
growth.
Supplementation: Use of protein powders, creatine, and
amino acids.
Recovery: Adequate rest and sleep to promote muscle
recovery and growth.
Goals:

Achieve muscular hypertrophy (increased muscle size).
Sculpt the physique through targeted exercises and diet.
Compete in bodybuilding competitions at amateur or
professional levels.
Muscle Gain

Definition: Muscle gain refers to the increase in muscle mass and strength achieved through resistance training and proper nutrition.

Factors:

Progressive Overload: Gradually increasing resistance or volume to challenge muscles.
Protein Synthesis: Protein intake to support muscle repair and growth.
Recovery: Adequate rest and nutrition for muscle recovery and adaptation.
Hormonal Balance: Optimal levels of testosterone and growth hormone for muscle development.
Strategies:

Focus on compound exercises (squats, deadlifts, bench press) to engage multiple muscle groups.
Eat a balanced diet rich in protein, carbohydrates, and healthy fats.
Track progress with measurements and strength gains over time.
Ensure proper hydration and sleep for recovery and growth.
Strength Training
Definition: Strength training involves exercises designed to improve muscular strength, endurance, and power.

Components:

Resistance Exercises: Using weights, resistance bands, or body weight to challenge muscles.
Progressive Resistance: Gradually increasing resistance or intensity over time.
Muscle Groups: Targeting specific muscle groups with exercises like squats, lunges, and rows.

Functional Movement: Incorporating movements that mimic daily activities or sports.
Benefits:

Increases muscle mass and bone density.
Improves joint function and flexibility.
Boosts metabolism and supports weight management.
Enhances athletic performance and reduces injury risk.
Cardiovascular Health
Definition: Cardiovascular health refers to the well-being of the heart, blood vessels, and overall circulatory system.

Factors:

Aerobic Exercise: Activities like running, cycling, swimming that elevate heart rate and improve cardiovascular endurance.
Heart Health: Strengthening heart muscles and improving blood flow.
Risk Factors: Managing cholesterol levels, blood pressure, and diabetes to reduce cardiovascular disease risk.
Benefits:

Enhances endurance and stamina.
Lowers blood pressure and cholesterol levels.
Reduces the risk of heart disease, stroke, and diabetes.
Improves overall quality of life and longevity.
Meal Planning
Definition: Meal planning involves organizing and preparing meals ahead of time to achieve nutrition goals efficiently.

Steps:

Goal Setting: Determine nutritional needs based on health goals (weight loss, muscle gain, etc.).
Menu Creation: Plan balanced meals with appropriate portions of proteins, carbohydrates, and fats.

Grocery Shopping: Compile a shopping list based on planned meals and healthy food choices.
Preparation: Cook and portion meals in advance for convenience and consistency.
Benefits:

Supports healthy eating habits and portion control.
Saves time and reduces impulsive food choices.
Ensures nutritional balance and variety in diet.
Facilitates adherence to dietary goals and promotes overall well-being.
Healthy Recipes
Definition: Healthy recipes are dishes that prioritize nutrition and use wholesome ingredients while limiting unhealthy fats, sugars, and additives.

Components:

Nutrient-Dense Ingredients: Whole grains, lean proteins, fruits, vegetables, and healthy fats.
Cooking Methods: Grilling, baking, steaming, or sautéing to preserve nutrients without excessive added fats.
Seasonings and Flavors: Herbs, spices, and natural flavor enhancers instead of salt and sugar.
Types:

Breakfast: Smoothies, overnight oats, whole grain pancakes.
Lunch and Dinner: Salads, stir-fries, grilled meats or fish with vegetables.
Snacks: Nut mixes, yogurt parfaits, vegetable sticks with hummus.
Benefits:

Provides essential nutrients for overall health and well-being.
Supports weight management and energy balance.

Promotes culinary creativity and enjoyment of nutritious foods.

Helps maintain a healthy lifestyle and prevent chronic diseases.

Weight Management

Definition: Weight management involves maintaining a healthy body weight through balanced nutrition, regular physical activity, and lifestyle modifications.

Strategies:

Calorie Balance: Adjusting calorie intake to match energy expenditure for weight maintenance or loss.

Physical Activity: Incorporating regular exercise and movement into daily routines.

Behavioral Changes: Adopting sustainable habits like mindful eating and portion control.

Health Monitoring: Tracking weight, body composition, and overall health indicators.

Benefits:

Improves overall health and reduces the risk of chronic diseases.

Enhances self-esteem and body image.

Supports long-term weight maintenance and sustainability.

Promotes healthy aging and quality of life.

Healthy Habits

Definition: Healthy habits are behaviors and routines that contribute to overall physical, mental, and emotional well-being.

Examples:

Nutrition: Eating balanced meals, staying hydrated, practicing portion control.

Physical Activity: Regular exercise, stretching, and movement.

Sleep: Prioritizing adequate sleep for rest and recovery.
Stress Management: Relaxation techniques, mindfulness, and resilience-building.
Hygiene: Proper handwashing, dental care, and personal cleanliness.
Benefits:

Enhances quality of life and longevity.
Reduces the risk of chronic diseases and conditions.
Supports mental clarity, focus, and emotional stability.
Promotes positive relationships and social interactions.
Stress Management
Definition: Stress management involves techniques and strategies to cope with and reduce stress levels, promoting overall well-being.

Approaches:

Mindfulness: Practicing present-moment awareness and meditation.
Physical Activity: Exercise, yoga, or tai chi to release tension and improve mood.
Relaxation: Deep breathing exercises, progressive muscle relaxation.
Time Management: Prioritizing tasks, setting realistic goals, and delegating responsibilities.
Benefits:

Reduces the negative effects of stress on physical and mental health.
Improves resilience and coping mechanisms.
Enhances overall emotional balance and well-being.
Supports immune function and reduces the risk of stress-related illnesses.
Mindfulness

Definition: Mindfulness is the practice of being present and fully engaged in the present moment without judgment.

Principles:

Awareness: Paying attention to thoughts, feelings, bodily sensations, and the surrounding environment.
Acceptance: Embracing thoughts and feelings without reacting or judging them.
Presence: Being fully engaged in the present moment with openness and curiosity.
Benefits:

Reduces stress and anxiety levels.
Improves focus, concentration, and cognitive function.
Enhances emotional regulation and resilience.
Promotes overall mental well-being and self-awareness.
Meditation
Definition: Meditation is a practice that involves focusing attention inward to achieve a heightened state of awareness, relaxation, and mental clarity.

Techniques:

Mindfulness Meditation: Focusing on breath, sensations, or thoughts to cultivate present-moment awareness.
Transcendental Meditation: Using a mantra or sound repetition to achieve a deep state of relaxation.
Guided Meditation: Following verbal instructions or visualizations from a teacher or recording.
Benefits:

Reduces stress and promotes relaxation.
Enhances emotional stability and resilience.
Improves concentration, memory, and cognitive function.
Supports spiritual growth and self-discovery.

Self-Care
Definition: Self-care involves deliberate actions and practices to nurture and prioritize one's physical, mental, and emotional well-being.

Components:

Physical: Exercise, healthy eating, adequate sleep, and regular medical check-ups.
Emotional: Stress management, relaxation techniques, hobbies, and creative outlets.
Social: Building supportive relationships, setting boundaries, and seeking social support.
Spiritual: Meditation, mindfulness, and practices that align with personal beliefs.
Benefits:

Enhances resilience and coping skills.
Improves overall mood and emotional balance.
Reduces burnout and compassion fatigue.
Promotes self-esteem and self-compassion.
Healthy Lifestyle
Definition: A healthy lifestyle encompasses habits, behaviors, and choices that contribute to overall health, well-being, and quality of life.

Elements:

Nutrition: Balanced diet, portion control, and mindful eating habits.
Physical Activity: Regular exercise, flexibility, and strength training.
Stress Management: Techniques to reduce stress and promote relaxation.
Sleep: Adequate sleep duration and quality for rest and recovery.

Social Connections: Building and maintaining supportive relationships.
Personal Development: Lifelong learning, goal setting, and self-improvement.
Benefits:

Enhances longevity and reduces the risk of chronic diseases.
Improves physical fitness, mental clarity, and emotional resilience.
Promotes positive relationships and social connections.
Supports a sense of purpose, fulfillment, and overall life satisfaction.
Healthy Mind
Definition: A healthy mind refers to mental well-being characterized by emotional resilience, cognitive function, and positive mental health.

Components:

Emotional Resilience: Coping with stress, adversity, and life challenges.
Cognitive Function: Mental clarity, focus, and memory.
Positive Mental Health: Optimism, self-esteem.